"*Bump On The* [Road is written by Cheryl] Barr about the impact of her husband Bill's severe brain injury, hope in the Lord, and their love for one another. It is a must-read for anyone who has a loved one who has suffered brain injury and believes in the power of God."

Nancy Markworth Brown, author of
Suddenly Your world Falls Apart- A Guide To Grieving Well-
Xulon Press

"If you have had to face unexpected tragedy, which puts demands upon you that seemed beyond your ability to handle, walk with Cheryl through her story. One feels like you are reading her diary. She boldly describes her innermost fears and struggles, beginning with receiving the initial shocking news to eventually finding overcoming victory. It is a testimony of depending upon God's faithful grace through much prayer and the promises of His Word. Her story is real and inspiring."

Marty Pfotenhauer
Married to Don Pfotenhauer, founding pastor of
Way of the Cross Church, Blaine, Minnesota
Coauthor of *Jesus, Where Are You Taking Us?*

"*Bump on the Road* is a gripping story about a family dealing with a severe brain injury. I could not put it down once I started reading it. I wept at the hard parts, I rejoiced at the small victories. Cheryl Barr has so articulately captured this challenging journey that she and her husband, Bill, and their family have gone through. The book honestly and candidly expresses the ups and downs of the journey. It brings honor to God and His "carrying the Barrs" for so many years. He will be glorified by this book, even as He is through Bill and Cheryl's lives."

Don Barr
Bill's brother and Bible Translator

Bump on the Road

My Husband's Recovery from Brain Injury

Blessings as you read our bumpy story,
Cheryl Barr

By Cheryl J. Barr

True North Publishing, Maple Grove MN

Bump on the Road: My Husband's Recovery From Brain Injury
Copyright © 2012 by Cheryl J. Barr

Published by TrueNorth Publishing,
6901 Ives Ln. N., Maple Grove, MN 55369
www.truenorthpublishingdt.com
Manufactured by Book Printing Revolution, Minneapolis, MN 55401

Cover design, interior art, and layout: Cheryl Barr
Photos courtesy of author
Editing: Delores E. Topliff, Creative Design Services,
www.delorestopliff.com

ISBN 978-0-9842291-6-1

Bump on the Road: My Husband's Recovery From Brain Injury
All rights reserved. No part of this book may be used or reproduced in any manner whatsoever without written permission from the author.

Published in the United States of America

FOREWORD

Cheryl's response to Bill's was the same most brides make on wedding days: "I (Cheryl) take thee (Bill) to be my lawful wedded husband…for better for worse, for richer for poorer, in sickness and in health, to love, cherish, and to obey, till death us do part…"

While serving as a church pastor and building a beautiful family, Bill made occasional short-term mission trips to India before possible full-time return there. Except one trip changed everything. A motorbike accident gave Bill a head injury so severe it nearly killed him. Their *Bump on the Road* changed them and their marriage forever.

Only strong marriages survive such tests. Weak marriages disintegrate on the rocks. Bill and Cheryl are not the same people who entered their marriage; they are better and their marriage stronger with Bill 90% recovered. And they've gained amazing wisdom in the process.

After gold is separated from the earth, most is heated and purified to reflect the refiner's image. Following the refining process, a small amount goes on to be hammered into malleable intricate forms. This book shares the furnace process that changed Bill and Cheryl Barr's lives from those containing much gold to those carefully worked to reveal infinitely more rare and precious beauty.

Delores E. Topliff
Author and President, Minnesota Christian Writers Guild
www.delorestopliff.com
Adjunct Professor, Northwestern College, St. Paul, Minnesota

Author's Note

The journey of writing our saga began unintentionally through sending email updates after Bill's accident. For several months, I wrote to friends and relatives daily about Bill's progress, or lack thereof. As the volume of reports took on book proportions, a few eventually encouraged me to write for publication. Initially, I brushed them off. However, reading every book about brain injury recovery I could find, caused me to wish for more information about a spouse's brain injury. Thus the idea of writing this book germinated and eventually sprouted. The first group I wish to thank are those who urged me to write.

Next, I thank those who advised me to lay important foundations for writing. One thing led to another and I joined the Minnesota Christian Writers' Guild. Attending MCWG, I learned about the craft of writing through speakers and workshops. Relationships grew, leading me into a critique group. There was much to learn. In the early days, I questioned my ability to write our story. My writing friends urged me to keep at it and affirmed that I could succeed. It's been hard work but, oh, so rewarding to learn a new skill.

I am forever grateful to a host of encouragers around the globe who have stood with us in prayer, affirmed our efforts, and helped in practical ways. This includes those who have read and critiqued my manuscript. We are blessed with an awesome family and a broad circle of friends who have supported us in many ways through the trials described here. A few of our heroes walk through these pages, but the volume would be much too large if I named everyone.

I invite you to join me in reflecting upon our pilgrimage through our life-altering experience with brain injury. Along the way, we repeatedly experienced God's faithfulness. Throughout Bill's recovery, I knew that he wasn't the only one who would end up different. I would change as well. No way would I want to waste this experience by returning to the same old me without positive growth.

I hope our story encourages those who are traveling through dark valleys, brings hope to those who feel like giving up, and helps those who have suddenly landed in a similar situation and wonder what will lie ahead.

This book is written to honor my husband, Bill, who endured the *Bump on the Road* without losing his cheerful, kind spirit.

– Cheryl Barr, October 2012

Prologue

April 29, 1968
College of Wooster, Wooster Ohio

Dear Lynn,

You won't believe what we did last week. Dave, Peg, Bill and I drove to Dayton to see Bill's parents. We had to cut classes on Thursday but none of us had anything pressing that day.

At 9:30 p.m. we left Wooster, drove three hours and arrived at the Barrs' home after midnight. It was late and I didn't want to get in trouble with the people I hoped would become my in-laws someday. We did it, anyway. Bill said it would be fine because his dad is a pastor and is accustomed to people dropping in at any time of the day or night.

I couldn't imagine doing that to my parents. They would already have been asleep for two or three hours.

Bill and I hid in the bushes while Peg and Dave rang the doorbell. Bill's dad answered. Dave and Peg introduced themselves, saying that they wanted counseling. He took them into the den and started toward the kitchen to get some snacks.

Dave told him that he had friends outside who also wanted help. Bill and I had crawled out from behind the bush and stood on the porch. When Mr. Barr saw us, his weary expression transformed into astonishment. "Well, I'll be!" He clapped his hands together. "You guys." He laughed. "Come on in!"

Mom Barr emerged, wearing her bathrobe and rubbing her eyes. "What's going on? Oh my!" She looked a bit embarrassed as though she should have been awake and expecting us. I love their spontaneity and warmth. They actually seemed happy to see us!

After talking awhile, we went to bed. The next day we had a fantastic time. In the afternoon the four of us talked freely with Mr. and Mrs. Barr about courtship and marriage, its problems and joys. All of us felt at ease with his parents. This helped make things more clear about Bill's and my relationship.

Bill's parents talked about giving love to each other 100% and wearing off the rough edges gradually, adapting into a harmonious relationship. By nature, Bill is more concerned about others than himself. I wish I could say that about me. I'm beginning to see that I need God's help to do what's hard for me to accomplish on my own.

After supper, we hit the road for Wooster. Bill and I became even more excited about relationship. If this leads to marriage, I hope I can be the kind of wife that Bill needs and deserves. It seems like he does all the giving and I just receive his goodness. Somehow, I need to find a way to give back to him.

There's something else that I worry about. He wants to go back to India where he grew up. Hopefully, that's a long time from now and I'll be ready by then!

Your friend,
Cheryl

January 26, 1999

THE PHONE RANG at 8:00 a.m. in my friend's cottage in rural Holland where I was staying. Still weary from spending three weeks in India, I finished washing up for the second half of my trip home to Minnesota. My husband, Bill, had remained near Delhi for two more weeks.

Marcia, my hostess, summoned me. "It's Jim Brown."

Why would Jim call now? It was 1:00 a.m. for our mutual friend. Couldn't he have waited until I got home to Minnesota?

"I have bad news for you, Cheryl. Bill was hurt in a serious motorcycle accident in India." Jim wasn't teasing this time.

My heart pounded as I gasped. "Is he okay?"

"They are doing surgery in half an hour to relieve pressure on his brain," said Jim. "This will spare his life."

Spare his life? I froze.

"You can use my credit card for a ticket to fly back to India."

Go back to India? Go. Back. To India. Could I face what awaited me there?

"We're praying for you," assured Jim. He gave me the hospital phone number and said, "Call back and let us know when you find out more from the hospital."

"What happened?" asked Marcia. Concern filled my hostess' soft brown eyes.

My legs turning to foam, I collapsed into a chair. "Bill was in a motor cycle accident." I remembered my Indian scooter ride two weeks earlier. I had clutched my friend's waist as she zigzagged us through a rushing torrent of wheels and legs. Black exhaust billowed from the busses and trucks that dominated the road.

I dug in my oversized purse in search of the phone number where my daughter was staying in another part of Holland. We had arranged to meet two hours later in Amsterdam for our trip home.

"I've got to catch Jody before she leaves for the airport." I looked at the phone and froze. "But how…" I had always depended on Bill to handle international calls.

"Go ahead and dial directly. It won't be much."

"Are you sure?" I would give her some money before I left.

Dare I hope that Jody would return to India with me? I was an adult and should stand with my husband no matter what. But I felt helpless. Thankfully, I caught my daughter before she left.

"I'll go with you," Jody said. "I have a week before I absolutely have to be back for classes." My daughter's words soothed my soul. I wasn't sure I could do this alone.

A last minute financial miracle had funded our trip. Now what? I couldn't let myself figure that out now. Bill needed medical help and I needed to go to him as soon as possible.

I cancelled our tickets home and booked two seats for the next day, hoping Bill wouldn't worry and wonder why I didn't reach his side sooner. Then I called the hospital and talked to someone named Chris. His scant information was like a teaspoon of water when I thirsted for a gallon.

Trying to visualize the setting, I remembered a visit to the hospital near Bill's childhood home in India. Walls were gray concrete and sunlight filtered in through small windows. Families camped out with the patients, providing meals and other non-medical care. It was dreary.

Now it was my turn, and I was scared. Where would I find food? How about moral support, especially if Jody left before I could? I had no idea what I would do. India was Bill's second home but a foreign country to me.

January 26, 1999

As I dressed, Marcia cleared her day's agenda. Her gentle stability consoled me. Forcing myself to eat yogurt and granola, I stared through the drizzle into the woods past her cottage. The heavens were weeping too.

"Bill has been through a lot in recent years, and now another thing," I sighed. Sipping peppermint tea, I described my husband's recent medical episodes. Vocational questions and financial insecurity plagued us as well. "I don't understand why he has to go through all this. I see why God allows this stuff with the proud and stubborn, but Bill? He doesn't need more 'breaking.' Of all the people I know, he's one of the most humble."

"I know." Marcia clasped my hand. "We can't understand why God allows such things, but I believe God most powerfully uses those who are broken of pride."

"Then God must have a really big plan for Bill." I blew my nose and sighed.

"*Ja.*" My American friend spoke like one of her Dutch friends.

We stayed near the phone all morning. I wrote an email update, asking Jim to forward it to many mutual friends. My initial adrenalin surge gave way to numbness and a mid-stomach knot. Marcia and I talked, prayed, pondered, wept, and shared memories.

Four hours later, Chris called from the Indian hospital. "The surgery was successful and they removed a sizable clot from beneath your husband's skull. After he regains consciousness, they'll run tests to know more."

"When will that be?"

"Within twenty-four hours we hope, Ma'am."

"Oh." My husband was unconscious. I was sitting in Holland fishing for answers from someone I didn't know. "Do you work at the hospital?"

"No Ma'am. I was with your husband when he had his accident."

Why did they have me talk to this guy whom I'd never met? Where were the doctors and where was Raj, the director of the Bible

Bump on the Road

school where Bill was teaching? I longed for *answers*. Would Bill be okay? Would life return to normal? Soon? "I'll call from the airport tomorrow before we get on the plane." Surely, Bill would be conscious by then; and they could assure me he would be fine.

Pastor Gordy called from our church. "Cheryl, we're praying for you. If there's anything we can do to help, let us know. Don't worry about the finances. It will get taken care of."

"Thank you! I really appreciate that." I breathed deeply for the first time in five hours. I couldn't begin to imagine how we could afford this expense.

What now? Bill had lived in India most of his boyhood, so he felt at home there. I had leaned heavily on my husband to negotiate India. For the first 26 years of marriage I had avoided India. Finally, I agreed to go for five months in 1994. Once we got him home, would Bill ever be able to go back to India?

To pass the time Marcia and I went out in her borrowed car. With umbrellas in hand, we toured the serene countryside, windmills, an old clock tower, a bakery, and shops. Under other circumstances, I would have enjoyed the day. Instead I was numb. I bought yarn and a crochet hook to occupy myself at the hospital. I couldn't fix Bill, but I could make a hat. We ate *pannekoeken*, (Dutch pancakes) in a neighboring village before returning to her apartment. The sky wept all day.

That evening I reorganized my stuff and washed the grime out of the clothes I had worn from India to Holland. When I pulled warm rayon pants from the dryer, something was wrong. My pants had shrunk at least three inches in length.

Marcia gasped. "I'm so sorry. This dryer gets really hot."

"It's all I have besides what I have on." I frowned as I looked down at myself. "My India clothes are in my big suitcase. I sure hope the airline sends our luggage back to India."

January 26, 1999

"Hey, let's try ironing them." She swung open the door into her little kitchen and unlatched a fold-down ironing board. I ironed while she pulled, one pant leg at a time.

"I think it's working!" Relief flooded my frame.

"Yahoo!"

We laughed. It was good medicine.

By morning, the length gained by ironing was lost. With pant legs flapping mid-calf, we left her cottage before daylight so I could catch an early train to Amsterdam. After hugging Marcia, I hopped aboard alone.

I claimed a seat by the window near the front, and a young woman wearing a KLM airlines uniform took the seat beside me. After chatting a bit with her, I attempted to read. Gradually, daylight revealed towns, fields, houses with thatched roofs, goats, chickens, multitudes on bicycles, and more. I remembered how I had ridden with Bill in the "First Class" compartment on an "Express Train" between two Indian cities. Stopping at nearly every village along the way, we finally debarked thirty-six hours later. I silently thanked the Dutch for their timely, speedy trains.

I was supposed to be home now. Instead, Jody and I were returning to India. Her going along helped take the edge off this bad dream. I hoped that the three of us could go home together soon. However, she only had a week to spare before starting her second semester of college. I couldn't ask her to postpone her return. I pushed the worries aside. It was too much to think about. *Lord, let us rendezvous quickly at the ticketing desk.*

Following a string of words I couldn't understand, I heard an announcement about trains closed off from reaching the airport. Surely I misunderstood. The flight attendant's blue eyes darkened with alarm. "We must get off."

"Can I go with you?" I didn't know what else I could do. Had Jody heard an announcement on her train? Would someone help her?

Bump on the Road

The train stopped at a station on the outskirts of Amsterdam. A second flight attendant joined us. We ran with hundreds of others up and down stairs and through tunnels in the terminal maze to catch another train. It emptied at a huge bus stand where thousands waited. All were desperate to reach Schiphol, the immense international airport. Taxis and busses came and went, quickly filling. *Please, God, help Jody and me get there and find each other!*

Eventually, we squeezed onto a bus.

At last, the bus stopped outside the terminal. The flight attendants hurried off and I dashed to the ticketing desk. Only thirty minutes remained before boarding time. Either Jody was hidden in the crowd or she hadn't arrived yet. I got our tickets and ran to the check-in line for Delhi. Anxiously I scanned the crowd. As my turn approached, I let others go ahead. I panicked. What would I do if she didn't get there in time for the flight?

Finally Jody pushed her way toward our predetermined rendezvous point. Jumping up and down wildly flailing my arms, I shouted, "Jody!" Her brown eyes brightened with relief. "Come under here. I have your ticket." She ducked under the blue velvet rope to join me next in line for an agent. Handing our tickets to the red-haired woman, I explained the reason for our return trip and asked if she could check on the whereabouts of our suitcases.

"I'm so sorry about your husband." She entered our flight number on her computer, and then frowned. "Unfortunately, your flight has been delayed for ten hours due to fog and pollution in Delhi. I'll see if there are any other flights to India." Jody and I looked at each other through tear-filled eyes.

The agent shook her head. "All flights to India are delayed. I'm so very sorry! What I can do is give you seats in world business class and give you vouchers for food during your delay."

She processed our tickets and led us to another woman at a desk who continued the kindness. She gave us food vouchers, told us about the coin-operated lockers on the lower level and suggested a short bus trip to the Corrie Ten Boom home and museum in Harlaam. After our frantic race to reach the airport, I was reluctant to leave. However, we needed a distraction to fill ten hours.

"Everyone is so understanding," said Jody.

"They really are." We clutched each other and cried again.

After regaining composure, we stowed our carry-on bags in steel lockers downstairs and caught the bus to Haarlem, telling the bus driver that we wanted to go to the Corrie Ten Boom home. He told us when to get off and how to find the museum. The brisk walk felt good.

A woman met us at the entrance. "Ma'am, your bus driver called and said you had dropped your baggage claim tickets on the bus. He left it at the Haarlem bus station but you should go back now and get it."

"Oh no." What would we have done if it hadn't been for the kind bus driver?

"Go ahead. There aren't many here for the tour so we'll just wait for an hour."

We walked-ran back to the station where we successfully secured our baggage tag. Then, for the second time, we arrived at the clock shop below the home where Corrie's family had hidden Jews from the Nazis. During Corrie's time, the clock shop was her father's business and the Ten Boom family lived upstairs.

About a dozen of us followed a tour guide through the small upstairs apartment. The guide recounted the story of how the Ten Boom family had been betrayed, arrested and put into concentration camps. Only Corrie survived. "Seeing how they suffered makes our situation seem like nothing," said Jody.

"That's for sure." I shuddered.

"Mom, look at this poem on the wall. *The Weaver*."

Quietly we read and pondered the words. I put my arm around Jody and said, "That comparison to a weaving certainly describes our lives, doesn't it?

She nodded. "The hard things are like the loose and dark threads on the under side, but they work together with the bright colors to form the tapestry of our lives."

After returning to the airport and before boarding the plane, I called the Delhi hospital. I wanted to assure Bill that we were on our way. Someone named Abraham came on the line this time. Who *are* these people they have me talk to, anyway? I wanted a doctor's report that Bill would recover quickly and completely.

"Is Bill conscious yet?"

"No, but he is stable," replied Abraham. "Don't worry, we are here with him and he is receiving good care."

Not conscious yet. My heart sank.

Once on the plane, we settled into world business class with its perks. More leg room and space were a welcome gift. There we sat, waiting another two hours before take off. Now we were twelve hours late.

"I sure hope we get there before your dad gets anxious about where we are." I sighed, then continued. "One of us has always been by his side when he's in the hospital."

"Yeah. I wonder how he'll be," said Jody. "I want to be there but I'm scared at the same time."

"Me too. I wonder when he'll be well enough to come home."

"I don't know why God allowed this to happen. You know?" She paused. "I don't want to sound mad at God or anything like that but it seems that God has a lot more planned for Dad."

"That's for sure. I don't believe he's accomplished everything that the Lord has in mind for him."

"I pray God turns this around for good somehow and heals Dad." She paused as a flight attendant walked by. "I'm scared to expect total healing and then be disappointed if it doesn't happen."

"I know. I have the same struggle. We need to give it to the Lord. That's all we can do."

January 26, 1999

Be positive, Cheryl. You can't let your mind go down the path of worst case scenarios, dragging Jody there with you!

"Thank you for your patience." A voice interrupted. "We apologize for the delay. We are now ready to depart for Delhi."

Jody explored the movie options on the personal movie screen in front of her. I closed my eyes to sleep. My thoughts went back thirty years to our wedding. The setting sun shining through the stained glass windows cast a warm glow upon us. Both of our dads were Presbyterian ministers. My dad walked me in and gave me away. Bill's dad officiated. Before three hundred people, we committed ourselves to each other.

For much of our married life, Bill had carried the weight of taking care of me. I was the wimpy one. The fearful one. The self-centered one. He had drawn me out of my bashful shell and had helped me gain confidence.

In sickness and in health, part of our wedding vows, echoed through my mind. Before his heart attack six years prior, Bill was the strong and healthy one. Through angioplasty, medications, and rehab therapy, he had regained health. He functioned normally again until a colon infection three years later that resulted in a colostomy for three months. I wouldn't want to repeat *that* ordeal.

Now this. My husband needed me more than ever.

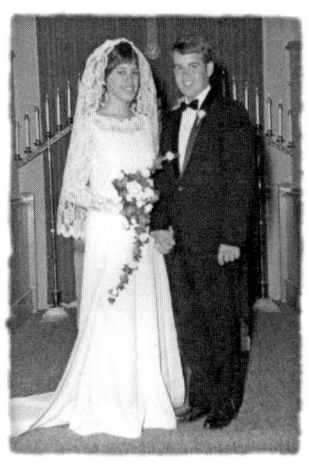

Where's My Husband?

TWO DAYS after Bill's accident, our jet descended through a smog blanket into Delhi. We hastened to the baggage claim area where suitcases and heavily taped boxes rolled past on a conveyer belt. Jody pressed through the crowd to grab our four big suitcases. I stood guard by our carry-on bags. We waited and waited. The crowd thinned to five of us staring longingly at the conveyor belt. Still no familiar suitcases.

I looked up to see Brother Kaushal, our friend, hurrying toward us. "Is everything okay? We've been waiting outside for three hours."

"I'm sorry. I was hoping you would somehow find out that we were delayed in Amsterdam."

"We heard. But the arrival board said your flight would be here at seven. We were worried. I must go back out. The security guard let me in but just for a minute."

"Our suitcases aren't here."

"Come, come." He spun around and marched toward a desk nearby. We followed. "Fill out these forms. I cannot stay in here. We'll wait outside."

I wondered how long I was stuck with my short pants.

After completing the forms, we found Brother Kaushal and his wife, Sona, outside. Horns blared. The sun bore through the thick haze. I braced myself against the pollution attack. India. Again. How long?

Sona, put her arm around my waist. "It's such a shame! I'm so, so sorry!" I wanted to withdraw. She was so mournful. Walk-

Where's My Husband?

ing between us, she grasped our hands as we followed her husband to the parking lot. Foreboding grew.

As the driver loaded our little bit of luggage into the large Jeep, Jody and I climbed into the back seat with Sona. Brother Kaushal took the middle seat. He introduced a tall, blonde American. This was Chris, the first man I talked to when I called the hospital. He was at the Bible Centre for ministry training under Brother Kaushal's leadership.

Turning toward us, Brother Kaushal detailed the entire episode.

It had been a national holiday so Bible school students and teachers had set out for downtown New Delhi to watch a parade. When there wasn't room for everyone in the Jeep, Bill and another man, Ingmar, had insisted on riding the motorcycle. Brother Kaushal protested, but relented. Only one helmet was available. Since Ingmar drove, he wore the helmet. Bill thought his Sikh turban would provide some protection. Ten minutes into the ride, someone in the Jeep looked back. "Stop! They're hurt!"

Both men had been thrown from the cycle and lay motionless. Apparently they had swerved to avoid a dog, hit a bump, flew through the air, and landed on the opposite side of the street.

Blood ran from Bill's nose, mouth and ears. His turban lay a few inches away. When no ambulance came, the students carefully loaded Ingmar and Bill into the Jeep and drove to the nearest hospital. By this time, Ingmar had begun to regain consciousness. He was admitted, but Bill's injuries were too severe. They transferred Bill to an ambulance, which dodged traffic all the way to a large government medical center. Because it was a national holiday, they refused to admit Bill. A third hospital had no space in its intensive care unit! However, a doctor there located a nearby facility that agreed to take him.

Bill's life depended upon immediate surgery, but someone needed to sign release forms and guarantee payment. Bible Centre staff intercepted Brother Kaushal before he boarded a train to another city. Two hours later, he had traversed Delhi's massive metropolis to sign the papers. Had surgery been delayed another half hour, Bill would have died.

This was too much to absorb, and my biggest question remained unanswered. *Will Bill recover?*

"I have Bill's passport and ring." Brother Kaushal reached into his pocket and frowned. "Unfortunately his ring was ruined. It was too tight so they had to cut it off to remove it." He handed me a small envelope. "They had to cut his jacket off, too, but it's with his other things at the Bible Centre."

I hoped the mangled wedding band didn't symbolize my husband's condition.

Instead of going directly to the hospital, we went to the center of Delhi. Surely Bill would awaken soon. Two days had passed since his accident. I dreaded going to the hospital, yet wondered why we didn't hurry over there before Bill wondered where I was.

After lunch in a Chinese restaurant, Brother K sent Chris with me into a large international bank to get cash. I handed my passport and credit card through the window's round opening.

"How much, Ma'am?"

"Two hundred dollars in rupees, please." I had no idea how much money I needed. Nor did I know how soon I could get more.

A few minutes later he returned with a three-inch stack of one hundred and five hundred rupee bills. Bill had always taken care of such details, so I was relieved that I had accomplished this independently.

"I have booked a room at the Y for your first two nights," said Brother Kaushal. "After that, you can stay at the Centre. We will go to the Y now. You can take rest." Another first—an Indian hotel without Bill. His name, William, means *Resolute Protector* and he had faithfully filled that role. Who would now? I silently thanked God for my mature nineteen year-old daughter. Together, we would manage.

We traveled a short distance to the hotel. "This is a good place. It is popular among international travelers," said our Indian friend.

The man at the desk handed me a note. "You have a message, Ma'am. Mr. Don Barr called. His phone number is here. He wants you to call him."

How would I call Bill's brother from here?

Brother K apparently read my mind. "You may use the guest phone in the room over this way." He led me to a semi-enclosed area where a phone sat on a small desk. "Tell the receptionist that you need to make a call, give him the number so they can place the call. They'll include it on your bill. You may also take meals here, which they will also put on your bill."

I tucked the paper in my purse, wondering when I would find time to call Don.

The driver and Chris grabbed our bulging carryon bags. We followed them up two flights of stairs. "Go ahead and freshen up a bit before we leave for the hospital," said Chris. "We'll wait for you downstairs. Take your time."

Our room had two single beds with a one-foot space between, a small bathroom, and a concrete deck barely large enough to stand on. I hugged Jody. "I'm so glad you're here!"

"Me too, Mom."

I sat on one of the beds, the typical two-inch cotton mattress on a board.

She began to fill a bucket in the bathroom. Water trickled slowly and stopped. "I hope the water comes back on so I can wash out my undies tonight!" She turned off the faucet.

"Are you ready to go see him?" I asked my daughter.

"As ready as I'll ever be, I 'spose. How 'bout you, Mom?"

"I want to be there but I'll have to admit, I'm nervous about seeing him."

"I feel the same way. When I heard about Dad's accident, I knew I wanted to come. But now I'm scared. He could look bad."

I pulled my daughter close and held her. "We should probably get going."

When he saw us come down the stairs, Brother Kaushal rose to his feet and motioned toward the phone room. "You may call your husband's brother now before we go to the hospital."

Though it delayed our arrival at Bill's bedside, I figured I might as well get it done. Amazingly, I succeeded easily. Don's voice on the other end was comforting.

"Since we're in the Philippines, I can get there in five hours by air. However, I have a problem. My passport is tied up in the process of extending my visa here. I'll see what I can do to expedite things, but it will still take awhile."

"I have no idea how long we'll be here, but I really appreciate your offer."

"Please stay in touch. I want to help if I can. I'll come as soon as possible if you're still there."

With that completed, we got back in the Jeep. This was the moment I both dreaded and wanted. What lay ahead? How would Bill look? What was the hospital like?

After dodging scooters, cows, bicyclists, and dogs for almost an hour, the Jeep slowed to turn into what looked like a shopping area. An officer in brown met us. Brother Kaushal sounded impatient as he exchanged a few words with the man. Finally, the uniformed man gestured toward the parking lot.

"Here's the hospital," said Brother Kaushal. Before me was an L-shaped structure with white arches that wrapped around two sides of a small parking lot. It appeared to be four stories tall.

Following our Indian friend, we ascended a gray terrazzo ramp hemmed by gray walls past another brown clad guard into a small lobby. I felt dozens of curious eyes fixed on us. *Sure wish I had my Indian clothes!*

Brother Kaushal stepped up to a large black desk flanked by a patient on a gurney and another in a wheelchair. A nurse wearing a white dress and stiff white cap nodded toward a doorway opposite the desk.

"Come, please." We followed her into a sunlit room. Two Indian men rose to greet us.

The man with oriental features waved toward two chairs. "Please be seated. I am Dr. Sing and this is Dr. Bose. We are on-call physicians. One of us is always here."

Dr. Bose pulled a large X-ray sheet from a file and handed it to Dr. Sing, who clipped it to a lighted board. "When Mr. Barr reached here, he was deeply comatose. He was bleeding from the ears and nose and vomiting."

I shuddered.

Pointing to the CT scan, Dr. Sing continued. "These are pictures of Mr. Barr's brain taken as if in cross sections. These are from when he first arrived." He pointed to darkened areas. "This is where there was clotting."

"See this?" He pointed to a curved dark line vertically intersecting a pear shape. "This is the midline of his brain. It is shifted over to the right."

He replaced that scan with another. "This is following surgery. See? The dark area from the clot is much smaller."

As he continued talking, his words got stuck somewhere between my ears and brain.

"Is Bill conscious yet?"

"Not yet, but he's improving each day."

"W-when do you think he will be conscious?"

"Just a few days. Swelling is slowly, slowly going down. When you go see Mr. Barr, he won't look good. Because of excessive fluid, he is bloated and bruised. His eyes are swollen closed."

At last the doctors dismissed us. We followed Brother Kaushal to the top floor where we approached a closed door. "Remove your shoes. Leave them here and wear these." He slipped on white flip flops which were by the door. Jody and I

Bump on the Road

followed his example. Then Brother K opened the door to a small bright room with two beds.

Two dark skinned nurses in white stood on both sides of a bed on which lay an immobile man.

Shocking. Worse than I had imagined. Bill's entire body looked like a water balloon with no distinction between chin and neck. Closed eyes bulged past the cheeks. They had shaved him head to toe. A white sheet covered his naked body from armpits to ankles. Cords ran from him to a sentry of machines.

Gingerly touching his exposed shoulder, I said, "Hi Bill." He looked as though he would explode if any more water entered his body. "We're here. Jody and I came back to be with you."

No response.

"I love you," I said before stepping aside.

"Hi Dad, it's Jody." She squeezed his hand and kissed his cheek. "I love you."

"He is getting better," said a nurse. "Starting to respond to pain stimulus on his right side." When she dug her fingernail into his left ear lobe, his toes flinched. "First he was paralyzed on both sides, but now he responds on right side."

Wasn't there a better way to assess pain than hurting him?

"Two of us are always with him," a nurse continued. "We take good care of him for you."

"Thank you." I hoped that, when it was my turn, I would know what to do.

"We will go now and let him rest," said Brother Kaushal.

I was relieved to leave Bill in the care of the nurses. Did he know I was even there? I wished I could rewind time one week and start over.

Brother Kaushal returned us to our hotel. "Get some rest now. We will return at seven this evening."

Jody and I forlornly climbed the concrete stairs to the dreary hotel room which matched our moods.

Home Away From Home

THE STARK small hotel room matched the chill in my heart. Jody eked out water to wash underwear and socks. "Will these dry better outside on the deck or in here?" Jody's question rescued me from remembering Bill's appearance.

I shrugged. "In here I 'spose. I'd rather not display my underwear to the world."

"Me neither."

After hanging socks and pants wherever we found space, we plopped down on our beds. "Jody. This would be... I couldn't have this alone."

"I couldn't have gone back."

I wondered if I would have done the same in her situation. This wasn't the first time Jody had endured hospital vigils with me. Yet, his minor heart attack and colon resection were easy compared to this.

"Oh Mom. Dad looked awful! It was horrible."

We embraced, wetting each other's hair with our tears. Then we slowly pulled apart and I returned to my bed.

"I wouldn't have recognized Dad if Brother Kaushal hadn't taken us in, would you Mom?"

"He was so...swollen. And those machines hooked up to him." I couldn't get the image of Bill's alien appearance out of my mind.

"Do you think Dad knew we were there?"

Bump on the Road

"Couldn't tell." I shrugged. "At least we're here in case it makes a difference."

"I think he squeezed my hand a little." She shivered. "I feel horrible saying this but I was so shocked by his appearance that I wanted to leave the room. It was hard to look at him."

"Oh, I know. I felt the same. We've come all this way to be with him and then to feel like running away…"

"It doesn't look like Dad will get out before I have to go back for classes." She finger-combed her shoulder-length brown hair.

"I know. I sure hope we can stay at someone's home where they speak good English." I dreaded being on my own. Alone. Waiting. Indefinitely. My future was shadowy, but what kind of mother would derail her daughter's career preparation?

"Something will work out, Mom. You know people here."

Could those we knew provide solace and friendship? I was stuck for who knew how long. Weeks? Months? Who would be my emotional support?

I looked at my watch. "We can go eat now. It's time."

"I'm not very hungry, but at least it's a diversion," said Jody.

After a dinner of chicken curry on rice at the hotel, we decided to look for the market that we had seen earlier. It was now dark and felt like bedtime.

A ten minute walk took us to rows of tiny shops and outdoor vendors with piles of merchandise. Expecting to find inexpensive Indian clothes, we found only jeans, shirts and sweaters.

"Buy this for your husband." A salesman pushed a maroon-colored fleece jacket toward me. "Very good quality. For you, only 250 rupees."

"No thank you." I started to leave. My husband. A pang went through my heart.

"Ma'am, I give you two for 150 rupees. Very good price. Good quality."

I relented, wondering if and when Bill would wear the two fleece shirts I now owned.

Having spent about ten dollars, we returned to our hotel with a couple of day's worth of pants and tops.

"Funny. When we wanted Indian clothes, we couldn't find them," I said.

"For sure. It's crazy how badly I wanted to buy western clothes when we were in Delhi last time," Jody said.

Brother Kaushal returned as planned and escorted us back to my silent spouse. Now that we were prepared for how Bill looked, it wasn't as hard to see him.

Upon returning to the lobby after a brief time with Bill, I recognized an Indian family waiting there. Bill and I had enjoyed our visit with them two weeks earlier.

"We live close by. Would you like to come stay with us?" asked Prasad.

"That would be wonderful!" This is what we had prayed for. Being from two different parts of India, English was the only language both spouses knew.

"We need two or three days to switch things around. Then, please come."

I looked at Brother Kaushal, expecting him to share my enthusiasm. His home was two hours away from the hospital, so we understood why he had not invited us to stay there.

He hesitated. "You should come to the Centre first. Then perhaps you can go to them later."

I consented, wondering how that would work. Hadn't he said that the Centre was far away and lacked public transportation? How would we reach the hospital? What about meals? If we used the Centre's kitchen, where would we buy food? Didn't only men stay there? Our presence could be awkward but we agreed because he was our guide.

Bump on the Road

⁂

Upon arriving at the hospital the following day, we met with the neurosurgeon. "Swelling should go down about two weeks after surgery. After that, when he's more stable, Mr. Barr can travel to a U.S. hospital."

"Will he be okay?"

"He will recover, but there was damage. Time will tell the extent. The clot was on the emotional center of the brain, but it's the least crucial area."

Least crucial area?

The doctor continued, "He might be irritable and aggressive for a while."

My husband has always been so gentle. Can I handle him being different?

"There were smaller clots and bruising in the area that affects vision."

"Will he be able to see?" *Oh God, help!*

"We'll know more after he becomes conscious."

"How soon will he talk to us?" *Surely God will surprise everyone with a speedy recovery and return to normal.*

"There's no way of knowing. It depends on how long his recovery takes. After the swelling goes down, there will be an indentation because part of his skull was removed. He will need surgery in six months to replace the skull piece."

"Did you save the skull bone?"

"No, no. We couldn't do that. They will make one of acrylic that will be as solid as the original. You need to find a neurologist in the States to continue care for your husband. Mr. Barr will need rehabilitation for about six months. He should be able to begin desk work in about three months."

I tried to imagine Bill's recovery but could not. I was only familiar with cardiac rehab. What happens in brain rehabilitation?

After this conversation and a brief visit upstairs with my non-responsive husband, we rejoined Chris in the lounge. "It helps to have you with us, but I feel bad for you sitting around all the time." *Surely this young man must wish he were doing something else.*

"I don't mind, Ma'am. I enjoyed getting to know your husband before his injury. Classes were cancelled because of the accident, so there's nothing else I need to do."

"Is there a restaurant nearby?" I asked. "I'll buy your lunch."

He hesitated. "I can show you where I got lunch the other day." We followed Chris across the parking lot to a small open-air curry shop. Except for a produce stand across the street, this was the only food in sight. Flies dined on dirty tables. Trash lay in reckless abandon. We bought yellow lentil curry over rice, chose the least filthy table, prayed over our food and ate.

Victor and Esther, whom we had met on a previous trip, arrived at the hospital after we returned from lunch. Having learned from Brother Kaushal that we needed clothes, they took us to a huge market area where I bought three Punjabi outfits that Jody and I would take turns wearing. I buried my short pants in my suitcase, hoping I wouldn't need them again. Now we wouldn't feel so out of place hanging out at the hospital.

೫ఎ

"We could use some words of hope right about now," I said as we sat on our hotel beds.

"That's for sure." She extracted a Bible and a devotional book from her suitcase. "Here's a list of scriptures by topic." She shuffled through some pages. "Affliction."

I retrieved my Bible. "Let's look them up."

We took turns finding and reading scriptures. The verses offered promises that God would restore the righteous after great troubles and that He was our strength through it all.

"If Bill, er Dad, isn't righteous, I don't know who is," I said. "Surely God will bring him out of this." We locked eyes and nodded in agreement that we would count on God's deliverance.

I must stay strong. If I dwell on Bill's condition too much, I'll fall apart.

"I wonder … should we take pictures of Dad?"

I shuddered at the thought. "I don't want to be reminded of how awful he looks."

"Me neither. Maybe when he's better we should," said Jody.

☙

The third night, we rode with Brother Kaushal to the Centre after sundown. I was hungry and wondered when we would eat supper. I sparingly sipped my water bottle, hoping that the Centre had filtered water.

Trees and rooftops rose above the thick cement walls lining both sides of the road. Pedestrians flowed along sidewalks. Bicyclists cruised past, weaving in and out between heavily loaded ox carts. Auto rickshaws (three-wheeled canvas enclosed scooters) puttered and bounced alongside busses, trucks and cars.

Eventually we turned into a residential area and parked by a new three-story house. "Here we are," Brother Kaushal announced.

The driver hopped out and unlocked the tall iron gate. He hauled our gear across a small patio, down a hallway past a motorcycle, and then inside.

Our hosts led us into a spacious room with two beds and an adjacent bathroom. A bowl of fruit topped a table between the beds. "Make yourselves comfortable," said Brother Kaushal. "Take some rest. If you would like a bath, turn on the *geezer* (water heater) with the switch twenty minutes beforehand." He lifted the cotton mattress to reveal a large storage area. "Here are towels and blankets."

Chris collected a toothbrush and towel from the bathroom.

"Is there a bus to the hospital, or can we get a rickshaw from here?" I asked.

"No, no. You will ride with someone from the Centre. Someone will go every day," replied Brother Kaushal.

"That will be wonderful." I was relieved to put off finding our own way for a bit longer.

The men went out to the living room.

I sneezed, sneezed and sneezed some more. Rummaging through my purse, I found tissue and antihistamines. "Delhi pollution must have caught up with me."

Chris knocked and entered with two cups of tea. A young man followed with a small tray of *biscuits* — mildly sweetened cookies. We sat on the beds, dunking biscuits in sweet and creamy aromatic Indian tea. The *chai* warmed my body and soul. As sneezes subsided, I began to relax.

Two familiar suitcases in the corner reminded me that Bill and Chris had shared this room. If we could break into the suitcases, we might find Bill's heart medications to take to the hospital. I wondered if it mattered. Everything was so different now. The suitcases' numerical combination was locked in Bill's brain. Would he remember it again?

I plopped down on Bill's smaller satchel while Jody pried the lock with a kitchen knife. Yea! The latches surrendered. Then we attacked the larger suitcase. Bottles of prescription medications, clothing, toiletries, a map of Delhi, Bible, notebooks, teaching notes, loose papers of various sizes with addresses and notes in Bill's familiar scrawl were as he had left them. The normal appearance of his things comforted me. It was as though he would return momentarily.

Bump on the Road

An hour later, we joined a circle of young men sitting cross-legged on a large mat covering the terrazzo floor. All were Indians except one. Wrapped in a wool plaid blanket, that man wore a gauze strip around his head, dark hair jutting around it. A fabric sling held one arm against his chest. This was Ingmar, the driver thrown from the same motorcycle as Bill. His broken bones seemed minor compared to Bill's broken brain. It didn't seem fair. My helmet-advocating man had gone without that fateful day. Why hadn't he bought one at a roadside market instead of expecting a turban to protect his head?

"I'm so sorry about your husband!" said Ingmar. Compassion intensified the shadows on his lean face.

"I'm sorry you were hurt, too. Do you remember it happening?" I replied.

"No, I don't. I was knocked out for twenty minutes."

Two Indian men shuttled in bowls of steaming hot rice, tortilla-like *chapatis*, and beans cooked in spicy sauce. We passed the dishes around, helping ourselves to the savory food.

A wall light broke the evening darkness. Ingmar explained that he was from Sweden but had grown up in India. I imagined that he and Bill had enjoyed sharing India stories. Would they have another chance?

After dinner we retired to our room.

"This *is* going to work." I looked at my daughter lying on the bed next to mine. "It's comforting to stay with someone, but I wonder if it's awkward for you."

"Yeah, a little. I feel like they're always watching me, though it's better than the hotel," she replied.

"I'm sooo glad this wasn't our first trip to India!" I shuddered. "Or that it didn't happen on one of the trips he made before I had ever come here. At least I feel like I know my way around a little."

"Me too. Wouldn't that have been awful to figure everything out without being familiar at all? To think you were paranoid about even coming here for so long."

"I know. I guess I was afraid because it was such a different culture. Now I know that people are people everywhere. All have the same needs."

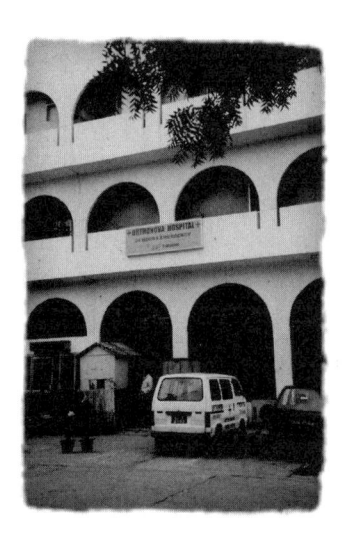

Our Every Need

THE NEXT MORNING, I was barely finished dressing when the Bible Centre's phone rang. A minute later, someone knocked on our door. "Ma'am, you have a phone call," said Chris. He directed me to the phone on a shelf around the corner.

"Your suitcases were delivered here to the house," said Bill's mom calling us from our home in Minnesota. Mom Barr lived with us and had just returned from her own overseas trip only to receive the horrific news of her son's accident.

"Oh no!" I said. "When I changed our flights, I specifically asked them to make sure our luggage came with us. Will they send them back?"

"Not unless we shell out $300 to send them cargo."

"You're kidding!"

"I kid you not! They won't do it now because I signed for them and they were *unaccompanied*." She sighed. "I was so upset! I'll send them, but they won't get there until Monday. It was my fault. I'll pay for it."

"That's ridiculous! We shouldn't have to pay for *their* mix-up." If I wasn't careful, my big-hearted mother-in-law would spend half of her monthly pension to send our suitcases back to India. "We're all set now. We went shopping with Esther and got some Indian clothes."

I hoped that I had persuaded her to not waste her money sending our suitcases.

While the guys finished making breakfast, I returned to our room and told Jody about the call from Mom.

"This must be really hard for Grandma, especially since she can't be here."

"It sounds like your Aunt Nancy is staying with her for a few days," I said.

"That's good. Otherwise she would be alone most of the time, worrying and wondering."

Peter, our nephew, also lived at our house while attending college; however, he wasn't around much.

Wrapping up in a shawl, I stuffed pillows between my back and the wall. Though only a few miles away, my husband, and closest friend, was absent. *Would I ever be able to talk to Bill heart to heart again? If so, would I remember all these things to tell him?* I picked up my journal and began to write.

> *Through Bill's suffering, God is working out the old junk in me. I'm leaning on God more, putting another first, receiving sacrificial love from people here; I'm becoming independent, but God-reliant. I've always relied on Bill in India—this is his thing, I' come to be with him. Now I'm here with him but in a totally different way.*
>
> *Psalm 34:19-20 says that we will have afflictions but that our bones aren't broken. Taken figuratively, I see bones as the foundation of our very being. Likewise, we will not be broken when our bedrock is in God. Lord, please reveal Your glory! Thank You for not breaking the infrastructure of our lives. Thank You for delivering us from our troubles though they seem many.*

I felt more desperate for God than ever before in my fifty-one years. God was my only hope. I couldn't remember being so helpless. This made my financial worries over the past 30 years seem like nothing.

Bump on the Road

After breakfast, Chris accompanied Jody and me to the hospital. I hoped I could manage on my own when I didn't have his help anymore.

Dreading lunch at the dirty cafe, I was overjoyed when a nurse asked if we wanted a hospital food tray. At least it would be sanitary food. An hour later, an orderly brought to us stainless steel divided plates filled with curried *dal* (beans or lentils), *chapatti*, rice, cucumber slices and an orange. We escaped to the tree surrounded deck to enjoy the pleasantly warm January day.

Chris introduced me to Hotmail at an Internet café near the hospital. I was delighted and sent several emails, promising updates every morning. Jim Brown would forward my emails to a growing list of concerned friends.

The next day, I discovered a flaw in my plan. The Internet café opened at noon. By then, people at home were sound asleep. It would take at least a day to receive their replies. This was just the beginning of our time difference challenges.

After three nights at the Centre, we prepared to move to Prasad and Beulah's home. Prasad arrived at the hospital after work on Tuesday. We filled the trunk of his little white car with our gear and headed toward his home.

As we talked about his work with computer software design, we dodged ox carts on the road. Trucks lumbered past, reminding me of our son Joel's boyhood constructions from his "spare parts" box.

The short distance to Prasad's took at least a half hour. We arrived in front of a white concrete apartment building. Prasad helped drag luggage up two flights of stairs. Beulah, his wife, welcomed us with her broad smile and twinkling brown eyes. Two young children bobbed up and down at her feet, intrigued yet bashful. Using one arm to pull a wheeled suitcase, Prasad swooped up his small daughter as he led us to our room. We unloaded our burdens onto the terrazzo floor. Two side by side single beds filled the room. A few books and toys were neatly stored on a shelf.

"This is your children's room, isn't it?" I asked. Again we were taking another's space.

"No problem!" He waved his hand and chuckled. "They'll sleep with us. They usually end up there, anyway."

Then Prasad showed us the bathroom. "Here is a bucket for your bath. Fill it here with this faucet." The wall faucet, about two feet from the floor, is a common feature in an Indian bathroom. "You've used these heaters before?" The foot-long coil immersion heater hung from a towel rack by a loose knot tied in its cord. A plastic spouted cup sat on the marble floor. Used for pouring water over oneself for bathing, this cup was standard for Asian bathrooms.

"For drinking and brushing teeth, use filtered water. We have filter in the kitchen." He motioned toward a bottle of water sitting on the marble counter near the sink bowl. "This has been filtered."

After we settled into our new quarters, Beulah summoned us to the living room. Insulated containers waited on a low coffee table between a couch and a single bed with an orange cotton spread. She removed a lid to reveal steaming *chapatis*. "Please, take and eat." She uncovered more dishes that held steaming rice and chicken curry.

"This looks wonderful." I said.

Prasad handed me a plate of cucumber slices. "If you are ready to leave by nine in the morning, you can ride as far as my office with me. The hospital is close by rickshaw from there."

"That would be great. We can be ready."

Beulah pulled stray strands of hair from her daughter's eyes. "Your mother, er, Bill's mother called this morning. She said that your friend's daughter works for the airlines, and they will send whatever you need to have sent back."

"Really?" I sat up straight.

"She wants you to call her and tell her what you need. They will also send money to compensate for the inconvenience of having your suitcases sent back to the States."

"That's amazing." This was even better than I had hoped.

☙

Two days later, Prasad drove us to the airport to retrieve the large suitcase which Mom had repacked. The connection with Mom through the suitcase was a comforting link with home. Besides, this was an assurance that God's hand was with us even to the smallest details.

Days passed more quickly than did Bill's recovery. I dreaded sending Jody home without us but there seemed to be no other option. Her classes were about to start.

A visit to the Internet café changed that. Jody's cousin, Joy, had sent an email about a conversation with Bill's mom and sister Nancy. They felt that Jody and I needed each other's support. Both Joy and Jody attended Bethel as pre-nursing students. Could Jody concentrate on school now, anyway? Joy had investigated Jody's options and learned she could make up some prerequisites during the summer and still enter the nursing program that fall. The nursing home, where they both worked, was willing to give Jody more time off, too.

This was beyond my wildest hopes. It was an easy decision for Jody. She didn't want to leave either.

Before going to sleep that night, I did what Bill had taught us to do–double-check the whereabouts of my passport. I emptied my purse twice, plowed through my carry-on, and dumped out my large suitcase. Jody dug through her things and I rummaged through Bill's suitcase. His was there but not mine. I panicked. Was it stolen? I remembered using it at the bank our first day back in Delhi. I was scared. What if I left it there, and an unscrupulous person kept it?

After searching every inch several times, I decided that all I could do was go to bed and wait until morning. I slept fitfully and awakened to a barrage of worries. I sat up on the bed, staring into the darkness. What if I were detained in India to get a replacement passport, long after Bill was released to go home? I struggled to reroute worry into prayer. This "little" problem was distracting me from a greater assignment. Bill was lying in a bed several miles from us with his very life and future dependent upon God's healing touch. He needed my prayers, not my worries! Eventually, peace returned and I drifted into a light sleep.

The next morning, Prasad called the bank. A concerned banker had guarded my passport, wondering what to do since she did not have an Indian address for me. I caught an auto rickshaw for downtown Delhi, profusely thanked the honest banker, and returned to the hospital relieved and grateful.

I was slowly learning to depend upon and trust God rather than to rely on my husband.

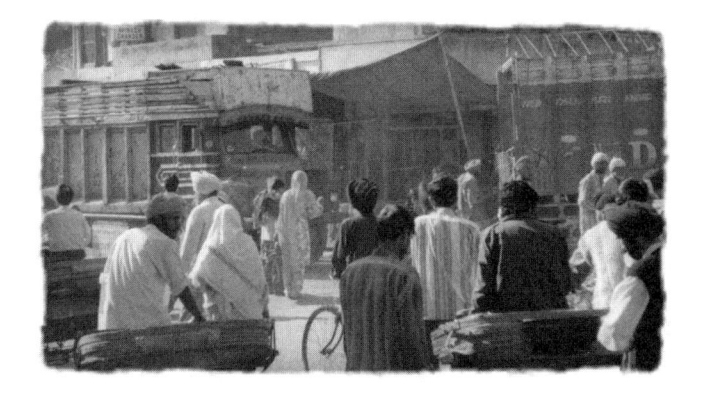

We Must Get Him Home

DONNING INDIAN CLOTHES for the day, I heard the phone ring. Shuffling flip-flops grew closer, then quieted as Beulah stopped outside our bedroom door. "Cheryl, it's Bill's sister."

"I'll be right there." Knowing that international calls cost several dollars per minute, I quickly tied my pants' drawstring and hurried to the living room.

"Cheryl, the trauma doctor at North Memorial Hospital still hasn't received a fax from Bill's doctor there." Nancy, Bill's sister, sounded concerned. "Faxes aren't getting through, and the doctor is never there when this doctor calls. They need more information to advise when Bill should return home."

"We'll get over there as soon as we can and ask about it. It's so hard doing this across the globe. I keep wondering if there's anything more that could be done for Bill if we were home."

Not only were our lives disrupted by Bill's bonk on the head. Mom, Nancy, and Jim Brown advocated our cause at home. I wondered how much of their time this was consuming. I longed to be with them so we could undergird each other.

The morning of February 1, Jody and I met with three doctors to discuss the most recent CT scans. I told them the doctor in Minnesota needed information. They agreed to do what they could to facilitate communication. They told us that the lack of blood supply causes swelling and that there wasn't anything anyone could do about the clotting. It would eventually clear on its own. The neurosurgeon said it would be at least two weeks before Bill would be stable enough to travel. They couldn't determine how long before he would be conscious, very possibly longer than two weeks.

When forwarding my email summary of this conversation, Jim added a note:

> It appears that the doctors in India don't know what to do for Bill anymore and would like for him to be sent home. We feel that the Indian doctor's reports to Cheryl may not be complete and that Bill is not in as good condition as we were first led to believe. Jim

Jim included an addendum to February 3 email as well:

> Bill still has not left India. With the 12-hour time difference the neurosurgeon was off duty, and the attending physician did not know enough about the case to release Bill. That puts us back another two days. Bill has been unconscious eight days now. Maximum swelling should last three to five days. Jim

After this volley of emails, a nurse intercepted us before we settled into the green couch for the day. "Three people called about Bill today."

"Who were they?" I asked.

"One was Bill's cousin, a doctor."

"R-really? Bill hasn't talked to him for a long, long time!" I didn't believe this.

"Mrs. Kapur called and about therapy. Dr. Gill also called."

As the nurse disappeared behind the curved desk, Jody nudged me. "So Dad has a cousin who's a doctor?"

"Yes, but they haven't been in touch for years."

"Who are those other people?" Jody lowered her voice to a whisper. "You'd think this was international news or something."

"Dr. Gill is an Indian surgeon that Dad's family knew when they lived in India. The last I knew, Dr. Gill was hospitalized at

Bump on the Road

Mayo after being in a bad accident. Dad and Grandma went to see him there. We hadn't heard how he's doing or where he is now."

"Who's the other one that called, Mrs. Kah something?"

"I have no idea."

Dr. Natan summoned us to his office. "I have spoken with the physician at North Memorial Hospital in Minneapolis. I explained our treatment. He said it would be best for your husband to travel home when he is physically stable. In about two weeks."

I began to wonder if we would ever go home. "Don't they want him sooner?" Certainly they could speed up Bill's recovery in the States.

"There's nothing they can do that we can't do here. He needs to be physically stable to travel. It would be too risky now. Your husband needs to rest, and the swelling needs to go down first. Two doctors you know called. I explained what we were doing."

Apparently, Mom had enlisted professionals to see if Bill was receiving proper care.

Though reassured, I longed to take Bill home. Was Dr. Natan's *another two weeks* going to turn into *two months*? Or *longer*?

As we finished our meal that evening, Beulah handed me a small paper with a phone number on it. "Mrs. Kapur called and would like you to phone her. Here's her number."

There was that name again. I had no idea who she was and didn't feel like calling anyone, especially a stranger. If she really wanted to talk to us, she would try again. It was late, and I still had to compose and send an email update.

The next morning the phone rang as we were preparing to leave. Prasad called from the living room. "Cheryl, it's Mrs. Kapur on the phone for you."

I put my bags down on the bed and went to the phone. Though frustrated with the distraction I was relieved that I didn't have to figure out when to call her.

We Must Get Him Home

In perfect English, Nita Kapur explained her relationship by marriage to the doctor cousin who had called. She said that they lived nearby, would pick us up for an evening in their home and offered lodging if we needed it. I was glad she had persisted. Experiences like this confirmed that God was watching over us.

From Prasad's living room on February 4, I emailed our friends at home who were waiting for news:

> Today Bill finally opened the least swollen eye in response to pain (pressure) stimulus on his ear and other places. We have been waiting for this. Progress is slow but steady. Today he also made sounds as though he were attempting to communicate. He has been moved from ICU to a private room with continued 24-hour care. He receives liquid food through a tube down his throat and now breathes without extra oxygen.
>
> I'm so grateful Jody can stay with me. She's a stabilizing source and comfort, a precious daughter! Today she rubbed the knots out of my back. This experience is forcing me to grow up. I'd always depended on Bill in this land, viewing it as "his thing." Now we are independent, yet dependent on our heavenly Father. Thankfully, this is not our first time in this country! THANKS HEAPS for your prayers, phone calls, emails, help and everything! You're all wonderful!

I held onto a gradually weakening thread of hope that Bill would suddenly wake up and be his former self. Isn't that what happens in the movies? Besides, God works miracles. Why couldn't God simply snap Bill out of this?

The next morning, February 5, Don called to say that he was on his way and would arrive that night. This was four days sooner than he had thought possible. Beulah put clean sheets on the living room bed.

Bump on the Road

Though I hadn't expected to need his help initially, I was relieved that he was coming. Not only had Don grown up in India, but he had lived in Asia more than in the States since then. He could help navigate whatever international challenges lay ahead. I hoped Jody wouldn't feel displaced by him after her sacrifice. I still needed her, too.

Prasad drove Jody and me to the airport. I chattered the whole way, describing Bill's family history to Prasad.

I remembered how vulnerable I had felt when arriving in India late at night. Eager cab drivers sat like vultures, watching to sock foreigners with a high-priced ride. No bartering over taxi fares or hotel rates late at night this time, thanks to Prasad!

A dazed and weary Don wandered out of the terminal. Though as short as most Indians, he was easy to spot because of his light coloring. I eagerly introduced him to Prasad, and we were on our way.

Don described his paperwork miracle. A coworker had advised him on how to expedite the process. By going to various offices, Don renewed his visa to the Philippines and then obtained a visa to India. In just five hours, God accomplished what Don had expected would take a week.

Could Don's arrival possibly trigger Bill to consciousness?

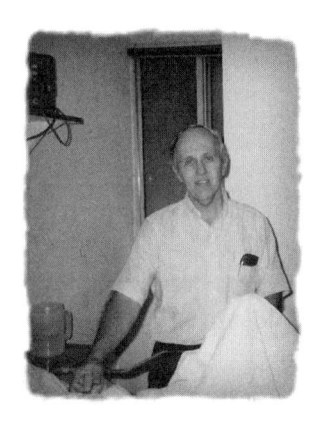

Ship Coming into Harbor

BILL'S SLUMBER flowed from one day into the next without any apparent recognition of Don.

"When will he start to respond?" I asked Dr. Natan. I didn't care if this question was getting old.

"We have no way of knowing. His recovery is slower than some, but each injury is different."

"Will he respond again…sometime?"

Tipping his head from side to side in Indian fashion, he replied. "Yes, yes, he will get better. I took my training at a Christian hospital in India. Missionary doctors came there to teach and work. One was the founding father in brain and neurological discoveries. He told us that recovery is like a ship coming into harbor, stopping at islands on the way to shore. Then the ship moves toward another island closer to shore. It stays there for a while. Slowly, slowly, it gets closer and closer to shore, stopping at many islands along the way. Eventually, the ship reaches harbor.

"Your husband should be okay for travel in … a couple of weeks, though there will be limitations and restrictions for about six months. I have seen such injuries before, and all have completely recovered."

"That's good!" Jody looked as relieved as I felt by these hopeful words.

After this conversation, we went to Bill's room. A nurse pinched and twisted his ear, checking the depth of his coma.

Bump on the Road

"Ouch!" Bill's first word. Jody and I smiled at each other. I felt guilty being happy to hear him react to pain.

"He has said *ouch* several times today, clearly like that," she reported. "He is getting better."

Two weeks had passed since Bill's accident, and he looked more like himself. The swelling was significantly reduced. He was still pale and had dark circles around his eyes. Though still somewhat bruised, his eyes no longer bulged. The swelling had diminished but not completely. He wasn't grotesque anymore. Nevertheless, he was still a specter of his former self.

ಐ

We sat on a wide concrete wall edging hospital deck and huddled around Don's camera screen to view pictures. Two gray haired men approached. One looked American and the other Indian. "Hello. Are you Bill Barr's family?"

I glanced at Don. He stood and greeted them properly with a handshake. "I am Bill's brother, Don."

"Donny! I remember you as a boy," said the lighter skinned man. "You and Billy used to run around, playing for hours. I worked with your parents; and this is Ramesh, also from Ferozpore at the time."

"What a pleasure to see you again." Don motioned toward Jody and me, "This is Bill's wife, Cheryl, and their daughter, Jody."

"We were at the Chinese restaurant in Connaught Place meeting with two coworkers. I heard a gentleman nearby say that Bill Barr met with an accident here. I knew Bill and Wilma Barr many years ago when they were working in north India. I could not constrain myself from finding out if this was the same person. So I asked the gentleman if he was speaking of the Bill Barr married to Willie."

"That's amazing," said Don.

Ship Coming into Harbor

"The gentleman at the restaurant was your friend, Mr. Kaushal. He explained it was Bill and Willie Barr's son. I said that I must see Billy. He told us that Billy was here." The man frowned. "We are so sorry. We will pray for complete recovery!"

Another day, as we sat curled up with books on the L-shaped sofa, two men walked toward us.

"Mrs. Barr?" A tall westerner extended his hand.

"Yes." I returned his hand shake wishing I didn't have to relate to one more sympathetic stranger.

"May I, please?" He gestured toward the spot on the couch next to me. I nodded.

"We learned of your husband's accident and came to see if we can help you." He introduced himself as the Regional Director of a large international organization and explained that he was in Delhi briefly. A mutual friend had told him about Bill. He gave me an address for his associate who would give us financial help. "If you need anything more, don't hesitate to call." He wrote his contact info on a slip of paper, wished us well, and left.

The next day I sat at Bill's bedside and looked up to see Mr. Narung walk in. Bill and I had spent a week with the Narungs earlier on this trip. During our visit, he had instructed Bill on how to wrap a turban Punjabi Sikh style. Though good friends, we only knew him as Mr. Narung.

I hopped up. "It's so good to see you!"

A faint smile glanced across his solemn face as he approached us. Mr. Narung hugged me sideways and looked at Don.

Approaching Bill, his face was grave as though peering into a casket at a funeral. Mr. Narung took Bill's hand and talked to him briefly. Then he turned toward us. "Come. Let me buy you a good meal."

We climbed into a black and yellow taxi together and rode a short distance. In the restaurant, a man wearing a white shirt and black trousers, led us to a long table covered with white linen.

"Please get what you want," said our friend. "They serve fine curry here."

A waiter appeared. "Would you like some *chapatis*? Or *chai*?"

I nodded. "Yes please."

Twenty minutes later, we were surrounded by *chapatis*, curried chicken, rice, and vegetables. I began to partake and then looked at our host. "Aren't you eating anything?"

"No, not now. We'll just have tea."

"Are you sure? You don't need to pay for our food."

"No, no, please eat. We are buying."

"I feel bad eating in front of you." Jody's chagrined expression mirrored what I felt.

"I don't eat when my brother lies in hospital," said Mr. Narung. "Please eat. You need nourishment."

Oh. Here I'm feasting when it's my husband that's in the hospital. Jody and I looked at each other. Then I looked Don's direction. I interpreted his look as "It's okay, don't worry about it." So we ate as our friend sipped tea.

When finished, we returned to Bill's bedside. Mr. Narung grasped Bill's hand. "Dear Lord Jesus, please heal my precious brother Bill. Deliver him from this affliction and bring healing and restoration to Your purposes for his life according to Your name, precious Jesus. Thank You Lord. Amen."

"He opened his eyes," said Don.

"Really?" I looked at Bill expectantly but my hope hit the floor. Bill's eyes were closed.

"It seemed that he responded to your voice," said Don.

Tears collected in Mr. Narung's eyes. "Bill is my dear friend."

I turned toward my brother-in-law. "Did he show any signs of recognition?"

"No, his look was blank," said Don. "Yet it was a significant step of progress."

Ship Coming into Harbor

"Yes, it was." I let out a deep breath. I hoped I wouldn't miss it next time. "It's the first time he's responded to someone's voice rather than just to the nurse poking and pinching."

Mr. Narung squeezed Bill's hand. "I must go now. I love you, brother, and will continue to pray for you."

Bidding farewell, he left to catch a bus back home. I figured it would be at least midnight by the time he got there. After a short night, he would teach math all day. I couldn't have done it.

"What a kind man," said Don. "He must think much of Bill."

"Yes, his home is six hours away by train, but he came by bus. Who knows how long that would take." I groaned as I imagined traveling Indian roads twice in one day.

"That's amazing. You have wonderful friends here."

"Yes, we really do."

The next day, Nita Kapur's husband picked the three of us up and drove us to their finely furnished home. Nita and her husband's extensive travels had included visits with the shared Barr relatives. She showed us recent pictures. *Oh how I wish Bill could be here, too.* He had talked often of his cousin and her husband Ashok from India.

I felt almost euphoric from the love lavished upon us. However, the shell of Bill reminded me why this was happening. If only Bill could grasp how many loved him. It would remove his self-doubt and insecurity.

Hopefully I can tell him all about it someday.

Riding in an auto rickshaw to Prasad and Beulah's, Jody leaned toward me and shouted above the traffic roar. "I was so excited when the nurses told us that Dad had opened his eyes and bummed that we weren't there. Today, when we finally saw his eyes open, it was a horrible disappointment. I was expecting him to connect with us."

"I was hoping for some sort of recognition," I said.

Bump on the Road

"His look was so blank, as though he wasn't even there. I hate to say it but I think Dad's recovery is going to take a long time."

February 9 Email:

> This afternoon, we saw more progress. When we entered Bill's room, his eyes were open. Until now, he's only awakened to ear twisting by the nurses. He's reacting now, pushing away the nurse's hand and saying, "Ouch." He is moving more, as though trying to get cozy. He looked at his left arm as if looking for his watch. He has begun to track with his eyes, move his head back and forth and make occasional attempts to speak. Tomorrow they plan to remove his sutures. Though open occasionally, Bill's eyes are lifeless as black marbles. I long to see their warm sparkle return.

A physical therapist started coming daily. She moved Bill's arms and legs in large circles, one at a time. "This will keep his joints from getting stiff," she said. "It is also good for his muscles and circulation. Mrs. Kapur arranged for me to come. He is still having basic responses only, reacting to pain stimuli. Conditioned responses will take more time."

I watched as the therapist and nurse sat Bill up at the edge of his bed. They held him up but released him momentarily. I held my breath, half expecting him to topple. Instinctively, he sat upright briefly without support.

"If you can, bring in some music or something to read to him. Anything to stimulate him a little," said the therapist.

We followed her suggestions. Jody positioned headphones on Bill and pushed PLAY on his cassette tape player. He responded by moving his hand to the rhythm and adjusting the ear pieces. When we read scriptures, he moved around more.

February 13 Email:

> This is turning into quite the story! If nothing else, I should write it for Bill so he'll know how much has happened. He continues making small steps forward each day. Today he said "hi" in response to my greeting. It's so easy to take one's brain for granted until something happens to it. Though mine has slowed, I'm grateful it works!

When going through hard times, I tend to grin and bear it. Tough it out. I didn't dare let my feelings reach the surface lest I were overcome. Though I reported factual information about Bill's progress, sending emails was therapeutic. I didn't grasp the depth of injury to his brain. Existing in a numbed stupor, I put one foot in front of the other to make it through one day at a time.

☙

Sunday morning I tried to talk but nothing came out. "Jody," I squeaked, "I think I need to stay in today. Would you mind if I didn't go with you?" I was soul weary and now had laryngitis.

"Don't you want to see Dad? It's Valentine's Day."

"True, but I don't want to irritate my voice by riding in a rickshaw today." I didn't feel like celebrating. "Tell him Happy Valentine's Day, and that I will try to see him later."

She frowned. "Okay. Whatever."

Guilt yanked at my heart. It didn't matter to me if I saw him. Yet, another part of me screamed that it *should* matter if I were a good wife. My daughter was disappointed in me. "I'll see if I can get a ride with our friends, Scott and Anita, in their car. They said they were going to the hospital this afternoon."

Bill had always been good about remembering special days. This year ... would he even miss me if I didn't go? I wanted to stay home and not talk for a while. If he happened to wake up for Valentine's Day, I didn't want him to wonder where I was.

Bump on the Road

I found Scott's phone number and reached them successfully. An hour later, they arrived in their new Honda. I climbed into the back seat between their two little girls. Windows were rolled up, blocking most of the road noise. Indian music played quietly. It was surreal as though I were watching a movie.

Though still hoarse, my voice worked minimally.

"I want to find a Valentine for Bill but don't know what to get." I hoped a visual would trigger something in Bill's mind.

"We'll stop at a shopping center," said Scott. "They should have something."

Scott parked and we clambered out. His long legs carried him half way across the mall area before he glanced over his shoulder at us. Anita nodded toward a row of modern stores. "Let's try this card shop."

Sure enough, amidst the racks of cards, I found a small, stuffed, red heart with "I love you" printed on it. "Anita, look at this, it's perfect." It was almost the size of my palm. Small, but not too small.

"Yes, that is good."

Purchase in hand, we left the shop and found Scott outside McDonald's. *If this heart doesn't joggle his memory, nothing will.*

"Did you find anything, ladies?" he asked.

"Yes, I got this."

"Cool." He turned and ambled into the restaurant. We followed. He bought an ice cream cone for each of us, which immediately quieted his whining daughters.

I tucked the heart in my generous bag as we returned to the car. In fifteen minutes, we were at the hospital.

Anita and Scott exchanged a few words in Punjabi, her birth language. Then she turned to me. "I will stay out here with the girls. You go in with Scott." Their little girls had quickly bonded with "Uncle Bill" when he had played with them a few weeks earlier. Anita wisely avoided subjecting her daughters to their unresponsive friend. I hoped Bill would be more normal by the time our grandkids would see him.

We hiked up the three flights of stairs. As we entered Bill's room, Jody stood. "Dad, Scott and Mom are here."

Snore.

I sat in the chair she had vacated, dug out the little package and mustered cheerfulness. "Hi Bill. Happy Valentine's Day."

No response.

I put the heart in his hand and closed his fingers around it. "I got something for you. It's a valentine."

He relaxed his fingers and the heart slipped from his hand onto the bed.

I tried again. "Bill, it's for you. It's a valentine. It says, 'I love you.'"

I let go, and so did he. *Why did I bother?*

I caught the heart before it hit the floor.

Would Bill be able to show love again?

I picked up my purse and croaked out a brief farewell. "Goodbye, Bill. I'm going to go now. I love you."

"Cheryl," said Don, "I wonder if he'll respond to a kiss."

Forgetting that my laryngitis could be contagious, I bent over and kissed my husband lightly on the mouth.

He puckered his lips and gently returned my kiss.

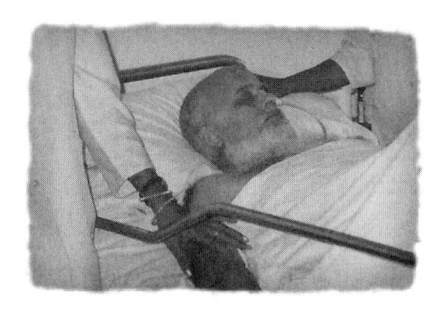

Repatriation

EARLY AFTERNOON SUN streamed through the window behind Dr. Sing as we gathered around his desk. A gentle breeze occasionally fluffed papers on a shelf behind him. Sounds from intersecting streets outside gave a backdrop of India style "white" noise. I vaguely noticed the putt-putt motors and croaky horns of auto rickshaws passing by.

"Bill will need physician assistance as he flies home. If he had a medical emergency, you wouldn't be able to help him. It would be good to get him home. I would like to go with you, if we can arrange it."

"That would be wonderful!" I had grown to appreciate Dr. Sing because of his compassionate nature.

"The problem is that it's very hard to get visas for our doctors. Often Indian doctors go there and don't come back. In fact, you will need two doctors because your husband still needs twenty-four hour care. We can draft a letter to explain the medical need and request attending physicians. Then you can take it to the embassy. Go first thing in the morning so you can get in the same day."

"We'll do whatever we need to," said Don.

"You will also need to go to your airline office to see about getting a block of tickets. I think we would need six spots for the stretcher plus two for doctors."

"Will insurance pay for this?" I asked. Provision for the three of us to go to India had arrived miraculously a week before we left. We had no savings account, and collectively our cars were worth a tenth

Repatriation

of what the tickets would cost. We could sell our house, but where would we live? If insurance refused to pay for Bill's return, I would be stuck in India until he recuperated enough to fly normally.

"Chances are that they will," answered the doctor. "We need a written request to your insurance company. It will be very, very expensive. We need to prove to them that it is a medical necessity for your husband to return home for further treatment."

Eagerly, I embraced the idea of going home but was overwhelmed by the logistics. Decisions and arrangements seemed endless. Pastor Gordy had said not to worry about finances, but did he anticipate all of this?

The three of us rode an auto rickshaw to the airline office in downtown Delhi. Walking through revolving glass doors, we stepped into a different world. Agents in blue sat on tall stools behind a desk that spanned the width of the room. The spacious, white surroundings reminded me of home.

Though the agents were sympathetic and helpful, their information wasn't. Besides tickets for two doctors, each seat removed would cost one ticket. Someone had to pay for Bill's travel and it wasn't coming as a gift from the airline. Surely God wouldn't leave us here indefinitely. Or would He? *Is this what I get for not agreeing to live in India when we considered it five years ago?*

Friends at home also investigated options. One negotiated with our insurance company. They would consider covering the cost only if transportation was certified by a bonafide medivac agency. Another woman tracked down a medical transport provider based in Calcutta. They would fly Bill the whole way on a special air ambulance. To start the process I needed to call Calcutta.

Again, I hiked across the hospital parking lot to the now familiar shanty labeled ISD, ICO, STD phone. I told the man behind the Plexiglass window that I wanted to call Calcutta. He

Bump on the Road

tipped his head toward an adjacent yellow walled enclosure. I got through on the first attempt.

"You need to fax release papers to us," said the director. "We must have a deposit of $200 to begin this process. Once we receive your deposit and paperwork, it will take a day or two to arrange for our plane to fly to Delhi. From Delhi we will fly your husband home. Payment is required before service." He went on to list the costs, a staggering $70,000 total.

"Isn't there a base here in Delhi?" Paying for a plane to come from Calcutta seemed like an exorbitant waste.

"No, we only have one in Calcutta."

Nothing in the nation's capitol, host city to thousands of internationals? It didn't make sense. "Will our insurance cover this?"

"I don't know. You need to provide proof that this is a medical necessity. Have your doctor write a letter to your insurance company. They will need to pay us up front. Since it will be a small plane, it will require several refueling stops. It will be a rougher ride and take longer than a commercial airline."

In spite of the paperwork, cost, and logistics, I was determined to get Bill home. This appeared to be our only choice.

I called Jim Brown about further arrangements on the States' side. He said that our friend had persisted with our insurance company until they agreed to pay 80% of Bill's transportation cost. However, they would not pay until after his return.

The transport provider requested a letter from family at home, seeking Bill's urgent repatriation. Then we needed visas for doctors as well as a release from Bill's doctors. Except for brief periods at the beginning and end of work days, doctors in India and the United States were not at work at the same time. Eleven and a half hours earlier in Minnesota, they were going to bed when we were already starting the next day. Besides, offices on both sides of the globe would close soon for the weekend.

Repatriation

Now that Bill could travel, how long would we have to wait because of paperwork? I longed for home and an American hospital. Our family, friends, and now insurance wanted him there, too. Certainly American medical practices could speed up his recovery.

I returned to the hospital and told our doctors about the call. "Oh no, don't do that," said Dr. Natan. "If you wait another couple of weeks, he can fly home in a seat next to you on a regular flight. We don't want you to have a financial disaster." How long would I be hostage to the "another two weeks" promise?

"Our insurance said they would cover it, and they want him to come home."

"All right, if you're sure you want to do it now, we'll fax a letter and the forms this afternoon."

By the end of the day, paperwork and deposit were sent.

Friday morning, Nita Kapur's call intercepted our take off for the hospital. I waited impatiently while Don talked to her. I sat down and sighed. We needed to catch the doctor right away to continue moving ahead in getting home.

I listened as Don told her about the Calcutta-based agency and wondered where the conversation was going.

"No, we haven't. We have been working with our doctors," Don told Nita. I studied his face. Was she also trying to get us to stay longer?

"Really. We did not know that." Don's countenance lightened. "Thank you! That would be most helpful!" He smiled as he hung up.

Curiosity overtook me. "What was that all about?"

"Amazing!" Don grinned. "She said that there is a medical transport provider here in Delhi. It's called East West. They repatriate foreigners who have been injured or become ill. She knows the head doctor and his Irish wife who's a nurse."

"Really?" This sounded too good to be true. "Are they dependable?"

"I'll call the American embassy to get their perspective. You and Jody go ahead to the hospital. I'll take care of this."

"Don, I don't know what I'd do without you!" I hugged my brother-in-law.

By the end of the day, Don had arranged for East West to evaluate Bill's condition. The doctor and his nurse wife examined Bill and reviewed his hospital charts. Bill slept through the entire discussion, oblivious to what was happening. Lying on his side facing the window, his hairy shoulder peeked above the white sheet covering his body. The doctor spread some papers on the empty bed in the room. His wife, Jody and I sat on chairs arranged in a semicircle between the beds as they explained the paperwork and expenses.

"We see no reason why Bill can't travel on a commercial airline. Medically, he is stable. He will travel on a stretcher, but this will require buying eight tickets. Unfortunately, the cost will be that of all seating spaces used. We will provide a doctor and a nurse to attend him continuously. They will take turns so that neither is on duty all the time and can rest. The flight with one ten hour layover in Amsterdam would be best."

"What will they do with my dad during the layover?" Jody asked what I was wondering.

"No problem. There is a fully equipped clinic in the airport. He will have a room where he will rest."

Perhaps home wasn't so far away, after all.

"We have a travel agent who will obtain tickets," the doctor continued. "We will try to get both of you on the same flight, too."

Though afraid of the answer, I asked, "What about the cost? Our insurance company has agreed to cover 80% within seven days afterwards."

Repatriation

"Don has already communicated with them by fax, and they agreed to send full payment within seven days." He explained the breakdown of expenses which he had written for Don earlier.

"Yes, that's the incredible part," said Don. "They let me use one of the computers downstairs to fax the insurance company. We can go ahead when there's space on a flight."

"We are also sending and receiving fax documentation from them," said the wife. "We have done this for fifteen years now, repatriating people all over the world."

"This sounds so much better! It helps to have someone right here in Delhi." Besides, the cost was a fraction of what the other agency was going to charge.

Paperwork completed, they shook our hands. "We should have you on your way within a week."

"Thank you sooo much!" I exhaled 18 days worth of tension. I could wait now, knowing we wouldn't be stuck there for 18 weeks or the rest of our lives.

As they left, I turned to Don and Jody. "This is turning into quite the story."

I almost galloped to the Plexiglas phone booth by the yellow building. Explaining that we had found someone in Delhi, I cancelled the air ambulance from Calcutta. They would not return the $200 deposit, but at least we hadn't paid more!

Thank You Lord for Nita Kapur!

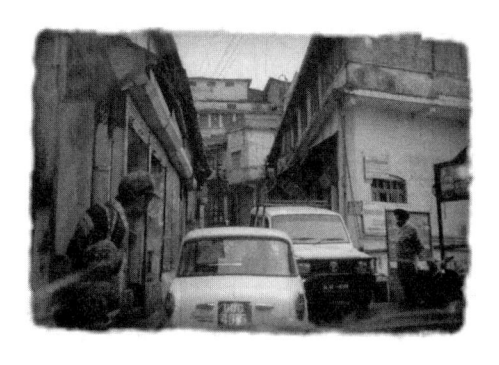

Home

FOUR DAYS LATER, Prasad drove Don, Jody and me to the hospital. We collected Bill's things while a male nurse aide dressed Bill in his pajamas. This was Bill's first clothing after his were cut off three weeks earlier. The doctor and nurse from East West arrived. Their efficiency and pleasant manner put me at ease. Brother Kaushal and a driver arrived to deliver us to the airport.

At long last, 10:00 p.m. rolled around and it was time to leave. The aide transferred Bill to a gurney and wheeled him out, down the elevator and to an ambulance outside.

"All of you have become like family." I scanned the circle of friends and staff. "I wish we could take you home with us. We'll bring him back to visit so you can meet the real Bill."

"Please do," the nurses replied.

Don, Jody and I hugged Prasad goodbye and left with Brother Kaushal and his driver.

At the airport, we exchanged goodbye hugs and checked in for our flights.

At last. Home. Jody and I sat with Don in the departure area. "Don, I really appreciate your coming!" I said. "I don't think we could have done everything, especially when I had laryngitis."

"I'm glad I could be here. You're quite the courageous women, both of you. You seem to have a good handle on things."

His flight was announced, so we hugged before he dashed toward his gate.

Home

At last, we were going home. The future looked shaky, but we would soon be home. At last. Our own cars. Our own beds. Family.

Things seemed to move along smoothly…or were they? An agent by the gate approached us. "Are you traveling with Mr. Barr?"

"Yes, is everything…"

"The stretcher was supposed to come on the flight that arrived from Amsterdam. It didn't. We need to see if we can borrow one from another airline. If not, we can't take him on this flight."

God, have mercy! Please let there be a stretcher!

"It would be horrible if they can't get him on," said Jody. "Who knows how long we'd have to wait."

An hour after we were scheduled to leave, we finally heard our boarding call.

"Did they find a stretcher for my dad?" Jody asked the agent.

"They are trying to adapt one from another airline. You may go ahead and board."

We hurried to our seats in the plane's rear. Two men struggled to Jerry-rig a framework that would hold Bill's stretcher in place.

Then the doctor and nurse entered with Bill. Once Bill was positioned, the doctor hung Bill's IV bottle and feeding bag from the framework above his head. Airline crew pinned blankets to the frame for an enclosure.

"Dad has the best spot on the plane!"

"He doesn't have to sleep sitting up this time."

"Maybe Dad will get better faster where it's more familiar."

"I hope so. At least he's used to American hospitals. Maybe they have more they can do, too."

"It feels so good to go home." Jody leaned back and sighed.

"That's for sure. It will be great to *drive* to the hospital. Even our old cars seem luxurious now."

Bump on the Road

"Welcome to the twin cities of Minneapolis and St. Paul. Local time is 6:05 p.m. Temperature is 29 degrees Fahrenheit. You may now unbuckle your safety belts and proceed to United States Customs and Immigration. Then go to Baggage Claim to collect your luggage."

Home. At last. I jumped up to gather bags.

A flight attendant appeared. "Please wait here until the rest of the passengers have deplaned. Attendants will bring a gurney onboard and take Mr. Barr. Doctor, you and the nurse will go with Mr. Barr through immigration."

Oh well. What's a few more minutes?

I set my bag down on the seat. "Cheryl and Jody, you will go through immigration, get your luggage and your husband's, and then go through customs. Then meet your husband on the other side where an ambulance will be waiting."

Emptying the humungous jet seemed to take forever. At last, the plane was empty. We waited. Waited. And waited. Did they forget us? I was ready to go hunt someone down when two men arrived. They rolled Bill onto the wheeled stretcher and we followed. Heat blasted in the gateway, masking February's chill.

At the end of the gateway, I saw Nancy and Mom with noses pressed against the thick glass wall separating us. Behind them were Jim and Joan Brown. We waved vigorously and followed the gurney down a long ramp into a bright room where our luggage sat alone on a conveyor belt. Customs and Immigration proceedings completed, we ran down the ramp to the glass doors into Baggage Claim where a little group waited.

"I'm taking your baggage to your home. Your mom and Nancy will go with you to the hospital." Before I could hug them, Jim had loaded our baggage onto a cart before disappearing into the crowd.

The gurney crew appeared. "Follow us please." We wandered through a maze of hallways and ended up outside of the baggage area where an ambulance waited.

"Jody, come hop in with us, and we'll meet your mom at the hospital," said Nancy. Longingly, I watched them hurry toward the parking ramp.

"Mrs. Barr, you may ride up here in the front." The driver opened the passenger door and I climbed in for my first ambulance ride. The doctor and nurse rode in back with Bill.

Upon arrival at North Memorial Hospital, he told me to go to Patient Registration and said that Bill would go to the emergency room for evaluation. Before I could dissolve into the comforting arms of family and friends, I was in a small glass cubicle with a young woman at a desk.

"Mrs. Barr. Was your husband in a motor vehicle accident?"

"Yes, but...."

"Please fill out these forms. Then you can go see your husband in Emergency," she said.

Somehow I completed the forms. A nurse led me through a wide doorway, past a long desk and down a passage between curtained cubicles. She whisked aside a curtain where Bill lay silently on a bed. A tall man wearing a long white coat turned to greet me. "Hello Mrs. Barr. I am the head trauma care doctor."

"We have examined your husband. He received good care in India. They did the same things we would have done here."

"Good." So they didn't have any special hurry-up techniques here, after all.

"We have a team of physicians who work together. Our neurosurgeon will determine when your husband is ready to have the bone piece replaced. Did you bring that with you?"

"No, they didn't keep it. The doctor said you would replace it with an acrylic piece."

"We can do that."

Bump on the Road

I sure hope so.

"We'll finish his evaluation here and then move your husband to the neurological floor. You may wait in the family lounge."

I hurried out to join my family and friends. Finally.

Our oldest son, Joel, and his wife sat together on one side of the room. Across from them were our friends, John and Jackie, who had recently returned from one of their overseas mission trips. Jody was between Mom and Nancy on another couch. "Where are Jim and Joan?" I asked, eager to see them, too.

"They took your luggage to the house."

I dropped into a chair next to Jackie, and she grasped my hand. "I almost hopped a flight right to Delhi before coming home from Eastern Europe; but we found out that Don was going to be there. I would have been there in a heartbeat if I needed to!"

"Really?" I threw my arms around Jackie. "What a friend!"

An orderly appeared in the doorway and told us that we could see Bill two at a time. I had already been with my silent husband. Now I wanted to hang out with my responsive companions. "Go ahead. I can wait."

Each pair returned with funereal faces. Though no longer grotesque, the form of Bill lacked his warm personality.

After Joel and Bridget's turn with Bill, their sad faces brightened a bit. "We waited to tell Dad first, so now we can tell you," said Joel. "We're expecting a baby in September."

"That's wonderful! Did Dad respond?"

"No, but we'll tell him again after he gets better," said Bridget.

"Dad kept urging us to have another kid, so I wanted him to know first," said Joel.

"He'll be really excited … when he finally understands. He's missing out on so much! I sure hope I remember everything so I can tell him someday. He has no idea how many people all over the world love him."

Jody and I went to Bill's room last. "How's he doing?" I asked the nurse.

She shook her head. "He just pulled out his NG tube for the second time. They really hate those things, but it's worse on them when they pull it out, and we have to put it back in."

"Poor Dad! That must really hurt."

The idea of rethreading the plastic tube through Bill's nose down the throat to the stomach sounded grueling.

"We need to have you fill out some forms," said the nurse as she handed me a clipboard. "You can do this in the other room while I put the tube back in."

"I'll stay and hold his hand or something," said Jody.

The nurse shrugged. "If you want to but it's not necessary."

Fifteen minutes later, I returned.

"He didn't like that much, but it's done." The nurse took the forms from my hand. "We'll keep an eye on him and restrain his hands if necessary." She set cloth wristbands on the bedside table.

Jody and I stayed with Bill until he drifted into sleep.

"I thought that would be a good experience since I'm going to be a nurse," said Jody. "But it was horrible! Dad, the nurse, and I were all crying by the end. I'll never forget it."

At last, we rejoined Nancy and Mom downstairs. With Nancy at the wheel, we enjoyed a smooth, calm ride home and rounded the corner into our driveway moments before midnight. We decompressed around the kitchen table before falling into bed.

Whew. What a trip.

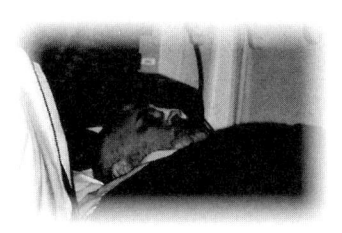

New Challenges

COLD CEREAL and granola tasted heavenly the next morning. After stowing dirty bowls in the dishwasher, Mom, Nancy, Jody and I returned to the hospital. Though the hospital was a half hour away, the absence of rickshaws, cows and crazy traffic made travel easy.

Bill had graduated from ICU Step-down to the neurological floor. We found his new room and lined up along the window sill. Medical staff started coming and going.

"Bill, I'm going to have you sit up for a little bit." The therapist rolled him to his side. "Okay, let's swing your legs over this way. That's right." As she talked, she manipulated his limbs accordingly. "Now, sit up. That's good." She put a three-inch wide belt around his waist, tightening a buckle at the back to fit. "Okay, we are going to stand up now."

Supporting him under the arm, she grasped the front of the belt with her other hand. She gently and slowly pulled him to a standing position. "Bill, now I want you to come over here and sit." She coached him through a slight pivot so that the backs of his knees were at the front edge of a chair by his bed. "Okay. I'll help you sit right here." She slowly lowered him into the chair. "Very good!"

During Bill's brief time sitting, she completed a form. Then she reversed the procedure, returning him to bed. "We'll get him up often to help his circulation and build his strength."

A few minutes later, another woman arrived. "I'm Barb from Occupational Therapy."

No more lying around snoozing life away for my husband.

"I'm going to evaluate Bill. We'll start taking him down to rehab after today; and we'll work on relearning self-care such as dressing, brushing his teeth, and so on." She talked to Bill a little bit, wrote notes and left.

Later another woman introduced herself as being from Speech Pathology. "We'll assess his ability to swallow. Once he is able to swallow, we'll start him on liquids."

The work of therapists was beginning.

"I need to access...," mumbled Bill as he pulled against the wristbands which attached him to a chair. It was our third day in Minnesota. When he couldn't get up, he settled back with a dejected, hopeless expression.

Staring at the floor, Bill shook his head. "Lord, have mercy."

"I don't think Dad feels very good," said Jody.

"Yeah, he looks as though he feels the way he did after heart and colon surgeries."

I made feeble attempts to converse. It seemed that my words plopped to the floor between us, repelled from his ears by an invisible shield. He attempted to stand again.

When the nurse helped him back into bed, I hoped a nap would help him feel better. However, he pulled against the wrist restraints, trying to sit up.

"He shouldn't get up because he's too confused. He might lose his balance and fall," said a nurse as she checked the bands connecting him to the bed.

I would never have imagined being relieved that my husband was held hostage to a hospital bed. A mere three days ago, he slept all the way here. I didn't know if I liked this new stage.

"It's a good thing we came home when we did," said Jody.

"That's for sure. Can you imagine him like this on the plane?"

Bump on the Road

ഔ

Friday, our third day home, I awoke to quiet voices in the kitchen. Putting on my bathrobe, I went downstairs.

Nancy looked up and smiled. "Good morning, Cheryl. Can I cook you some eggs?"

"Sure, but I'm not in any hurry. Feed yourselves first."

Mark, Nancy's husband, stood and engulfed me in a hug. My arms barely reached around half of his large chest. "Hi Cheryl."

Mom patted the tea pot. "Nancy made some Red Rose tea. I'll pour you some."

"Sounds good. Thanks."

"I'm taking Nancy home with me later today," said Mark as he pulled his wife closer. "I need her there."

Nancy giggled. "He's lost without me around."

"Aw come on. That's not true, though a whole month without you is tough." He tickled her as she refilled his coffee cup.

"Thanks for sharing your wife with us."

"That's what family is all about."

Nancy reached for a stack of notebooks and file folders on the table. "Before we leave, we need to go over some things. Mom and I were on the phone while you were in India. Nonstop."

"It rang constantly. We couldn't get anything done." Mom sighed. "It's a good thing there were two of us here."

"When we weren't talking to hospital or insurance people, we were getting calls from other people. You sure have lots of friends!" Nancy took a spiral notebook from the stack.

Mom fanned the pages of a small spiral pad. "At first we used my little everything notebook, but that filled up too fast."

"We decided that we needed a system." Nancy opened a 3-ring binder. "Copies of all your emails are in here." She picked up a file folder. "This has all your income tax stuff."

Oh. I had forgotten about that. Bill usually worked on taxes with Dave, an accountant friend.

"Dave said he would help you with your taxes." Nancy opened a spiral notebook. "We started recording phone conversations in here because we were grabbing for slips of paper to write on. Then we would lose those. At least, it's all in one place now."

I hoped I could manage now.

Nancy clasped my hand and looked at me tenderly. "We won't stop praying for you and for Bill. We love you guys. Lots."

"Thanks for everything," I said. "I had no idea how complicated things were on this end."

"He's my dear brother. Thank you for all you're doing to take care of him." Nancy pulled me into a hug.

When we arrived in Bill's room, our friend John was there. Clutching his Bible to his chest, John sat on the edge of Bill's bed.

"I've been reading scripture to Bill," said John. "He even said *amen* and *hallelujah* several times."

"That's cool," said Jody.

"His brain was injured, but not his spirit." John said.

Bill looked up, took my hand, and then bowed his head. The others followed his cue so that we formed a small circle holding hands. "Father," Bill prayed, "thank You for these people. Thank You for this opportunity. Please anoint us, direct us, and give us the strategy for reaching these people in Jesus' name."

I wondered what Bill saw in his mind's eye when he prayed. Were we crowded into an Indian village home? Or standing before a congregation?

I looked at the other bed in the room. Bill's roommate was in a chair in the hallway, swearing at everyone who walked by.

"I wish Bill could have a different roommate." I whispered.

Bill had something else on his mind. "I wonder when they'll bring my lunch."

Bump on the Road

Oh. I looked at Mom. She shrugged, grabbed Bill's hand, and talked as if to redirect his thoughts.

After Bill dozed off, Mom left with John. Jody and I remained.

By the time we arrived home later, it had been dark for several hours. Mom was in the kitchen, emptying the dishwasher. "There you are, you poor things. Aren't you exhausted?"

"Jet lag hit about the time we were halfway home." Jody kicked off her shoes by the door. "I'm famished now."

"Someone brought a meal. It's in the oven on warm, so come eat." Mom opened the oven. "Kathy from church is arranging meals for us. Isn't that wonderful? I told her that it's not necessary because I'm here, but they insist."

Three place settings were on the table. I looked at Mom. "Haven't you eaten yet?"

"No. I wanted to wait. I wasn't really hungry until now."

After feasting on chicken casserole, I looked at the clock and winced. "It's already nine thirty. I should send an email update, but I'm exhausted. I'll wait until morning."

The next morning Jim Brown called. "Hey you, where was that update last night? I waited up, but finally went to bed at one."

"Oh no." I felt terrible. "You didn't need to do that."

"Oh yes I did. Next time, call so I don't wait up."

"I'm sorry, Jim."

"Well, okay. This time." Jim chuckled. "I guess you need your beauty rest."

"I'll go write one right now."

"You'd better. You know, I charge extra." He laughed again.

Beneath Jim's fake sternness was a heart of gold.

☙

Our first time back at church started out like a cappuccino break after six hours on the road. Hugs from friends energized me,

New Challenges

and the worship songs lifted my spirit. I wept when we sang about being a vessel shaped by God for His purposes. I felt like a lump of clay on a potter's wheel, being reshaped from the inside out.

Then Pastor Gordy spread his notes and Bible on top of the podium. "I feel I'm supposed to do a series on marriage."

I moaned quietly and looked at Mom. She grasped my hand and squeezed it.

"One of the most important keys to a good marriage is good communication," Pastor continued.

Right. *What about when your husband can't talk to you?* I looked around at couples in the congregation. I knew that one couple was filing for divorce. *What could be any harder than what I'm going through? At least they can talk to each other.*

Hiding behind the tall man seated in front of me, I closed my eyes for a little nap. Instead of sleeping, I formed a plan. We would leave early or skip church for a few Sundays until Pastor was finished with this series.

After the service my friend, Marilee, grasped my hand. "We found out about Bill's accident at the Saturday women's breakfast. Jana told us. But we had no idea how serious it was. On Sunday, the next day, Pastor Gordy announced it," Marilee continued. "Colleen dashed up to the front and grabbed the mic. She said that this is really, really serious and that we need to intercede for Bill's life. The burden was so heavy on her. She dropped to the floor and cried out to God. The rest of us joined her in praying."

With this kind of prayer, Bill has to get well. But it's sure taking a long time.

❧

Soon after the doctor left the room, a petite brunette entered. She introduced herself as Julie, the social worker. My mind flashed back to a conversation with my sister who had been a social worker for brain-injured people in another city. I had struggled to understand her role. Now I was about to grasp it.

"I would like to get some information from you about what Bill was like before his accident," said Julie. "This gives us a better feel for what we can expect for recovery."

Pen in hand, she prepared to write. "How much education did he have?"

"He went to college and then three years of seminary."

"Good. We find that the more education a person has, the better the recovery. Tell me about his interests."

I looked toward the window and scratched my head. "He likes people. He was doing some remodeling and carpentry projects for others before his accident. When we were first married, he dragged me into some big creative projects. He designed a tent that went on a roof rack on top of our car."

"Really! Did you sleep in it up there?"

"Yes. We used a step ladder to get in."

"How cool. What else did he do?"

"We made a kayak from a kit which could seat four people."

"He sounds really talented."

"He's made lots of things but prefers being with people."

"Thanks for the info. This is helpful. We'll do what we can to steer him in these ways, though we have no way of knowing how much of this ability he'll recover. Personalities often change from brain injury, too. Sometimes angry people become mellow."

"Bill was one of the nicest, kindest guys around."

"We hope that he'll be that again."

∽

A neurologist stood at Bill's bedside, looking at the tube threaded through Bill's nose and throat to his stomach. "We would like to do a simple surgery and insert a feeding tube. It's important to keep his calorie and protein intake up. He needs better nourishment than we can give him through the NG tube."

"Can't we wait a little longer?" A stomach tube sounded too permanent. He had changed significantly since our flight home a week earlier.

"He isn't ready to take food by mouth. He could choke on it."

"How do they determine when he's ready?" Mom asked.

"The speech pathologist evaluates him periodically. Her report indicates that she tried giving him a little bit of crushed ice but he spit it back out. We are stretching things by using the NG this long. It's not intended for long term. Besides, he tends to pull it out. Don't worry. When he no longer needs the tube, it can be removed very simply."

We agreed to surgery on the following day.

Without the tube in his nose, Bill looked more normal. An eight inch wide band with Velcro fasteners was around his waist, covering the quarter inch thick, eighteen inch long tube inserted in his belly. How long would it take for him to discover this new intrusion into his body?

As was becoming a habit before going to bed that night, I descended to Bill's little office that had been carved out of a corner of the basement. There I booted up the laptop to check email and send an update about Bill's feeding tube.

> Bill converses quite a bit, though it's mostly about the world in his own mind. It reminds me of when he's talking in his sleep. As we get impatient with the process, we remind ourselves of the small but significant steps forward we see daily. Today, he said "Hi Mom" when he saw his mom though he called Jody "Josh" later in the day. His awareness shifts as often as Minnesota weather. Fear about the future stalks about, but God reminds us daily that He gives grace one day at a time.

Bump on the Road

The following day, social worker Julie returned. "We decided to try Bill on the rehab floor," said social worker Julie. "He has a good family support, and that's important for recovery. Upstairs in Rehab, patients wear clothes since we're trying to create more of a normal environment. Could you bring some loose-fitting clothes for Bill tomorrow?"

"Sure."

"Come. I'll take you up there and show you around."

As we rode the elevator up two floors, she talked. "On the rehab floor, the environment is less hospital-like. Family members and friends are encouraged to spend time with the patient. He will be in a room like this with one roommate."

Following her past the nurse station, we went to the opposite end of a long hall where we turned into a room overlooking a helicopter pad for air lifts. "This is the family lounge. You may bring your food and heat it up so that you can spend time with your family member. We have games here and this info about brain injury. You can bring in family photos. Label them so we can help him remember people in his life."

Back in the hallway, Julie stopped by large charts on the wall. "These describe the typical stages of recovery, ranging from one to ten with level one being in a coma."

"What level do you think he's at now?"

"He's probably somewhere between levels two and three where he's beginning to respond minimally. Stage ten is full recovery where they return to work and normal life."

"How long does that take?" That seemed impossible now.

"Since each injury is different, we can't say how long or how fully he'll recover. He will get better, but the brain heals slowly." She touched my arm lightly. "Be sure to take care of yourselves. This process takes awhile, and we want to make sure you get enough rest."

God wouldn't stop halfway, would He?

Rehabilitation

WAITING in the family lounge, I recognized a middle-aged couple from earlier. "What brings you here?"

"Our son, Matt, rolled his car two weeks ago. It was horrible." Her eyes glistened. "He was severely injured. He had cardiac arrest, and it didn't look like he would make it. In fact, his vital signs had stopped. He was pronounced dead and placed in a body bag."

I leaned forward.

"Then someone remembered he was supposed to do a blood test, so he went back." The mom uncoiled the tissue in her hand.

As she blew her nose, the man continued. "The guy started doing the test, and Matt opened his eyes! He checked Matt's pulse and discovered that Matthew's heart was beating."

"Wow!" I couldn't imagine how I would have felt if this had been my son.

"It's a miracle," said the couple in unison.

"That's for sure." I thought about Bill, lying motionless for three weeks. "How is he now?"

"He's getting better," said the man. "They have started getting him up, and he has gained enough strength to walk down the hall and back to his room."

"He started talking a few days ago, but he doesn't remember much yet." As she spoke, the mom pulled a new tissue from her pocket.

"That's amazing." Two weeks ago he was pronounced dead, and now he's walking and talking? "Someone must have been praying for him."

"We called our pastor right away and he got the whole church praying." He looked at his wife as she nodded.

If God can raise someone from the dead, He can bring Bill back. I took a deep breath as my hope level went up a notch.

"Thanks for telling us about your son."

We excused ourselves to go see if Bill was situated in his new room on the rehab floor. Jody grabbed the small suitcase between us. "It will be good to see Dad in regular clothes again."

"That's for sure. It feels like a sign of progress."

A nurse in brightly colored scrubs greeted us with a smile. "You may put his things into these drawers and here's a closet. It'll make it a tad bit homier for him."

Bill strained against the bands holding him in bed. I sat on the bed and held his hand, hoping to calm him. Formerly he thrived on affection. Now I was like another cloth restraint.

I looked at the metal bed rail inches from his head and remembered that a nurse had taped a pillow to it in his previous room. "Shouldn't he have some padding there so he doesn't hurt himself on the rail if he hits it?"

"I'll go get a cover." The nurse left and returned with a nylon stretchy piece that fit over the bed rail like a sock. She taped it on. "We have a high staff to patient ratio on this floor. Someone keeps an eye on our more agitated patients all the time."

Even so, I wondered if this was enough protection. Bill flopped in bed like a hooked walleye.

"This is stage three in the recovery scale." The nurse patted my hand that rested on Bill's bed rail. "He'll eventually pull through it."

"Will the next stage be easier?" I asked.

"He'll still be confused, but it should be easier because he'll start to understand a bit."

"Can we take him in the wheelchair around the hospital?"

"Sure, that might help distract him."

The nurse helped load Bill into a chair, and I pushed him to the end of the hall onto the elevator. On the main floor, we went to the lobby.

"Dad, let's go look at the fish." Jody walked at his side as I pushed.

Standing by the large aquarium, I pointed to the multitude of color swimming around. "Look at all the colorful fish, Bill."

His gaze remained downward. Then he tried to stand up. Jody turned his chair to face the fish tank. "See the fish, Dad?"

He lifted his face slightly. When he attempted to stand again, we moved on. As long as we kept moving, he stayed seated.

"I wonder if he can see the fish," said Jody. "Remember, in India they said his vision might be affected?"

"I hadn't thought of that." I waved my hand in front of his face. He blinked. "He saw that." I was relieved.

After a few more loops around the lobby, we returned Bill to his room. A nurse appeared as we rolled him through the doorway. "I'm going to take your temperature, Bill." She pulled a thermometer from its pouch.

"*Tek ha*," Bill mumbled.

"He still thinks he's in India," Jody said.

"Oh?" Bill's nurse looked at me quizzically.

"*Tek ha* means *okay* in Punjabi."

"Really. Does he use it often?" the nurse asked.

"Yes, we hear him say a few words here and there."

"That's helpful to know. We thought he was making up words. Would you write some of the words down for us?" She handed me a piece of paper.

Jody and I wrote words we remembered. After dozing ten minutes, Bill resumed flopping.

Bump on the Road

An aide arrived. "Bill, we're going to take you downstairs for some therapy."

Bill glanced up momentarily.

"Good!" I said, hoping she was more successful at engaging his attention.

The aide invited us to go along, so Jody and I followed them seven floors down on the elevator to the bowels of the hospital.

A cheerful woman, whom I recognized from the stream of therapists the first day, met us. "Hello Bill." Bill stared blankly at the woman's feet. "My name is Barb. Is this your wife and daughter?"

No response.

"Let's play some games." She set a peg on the floor a short distance from Bill's wheelchair. Then she handed him some rings. He let them drop.

"We're going to play ring toss. Let's pick up this ring and throw it over there and see if you can get it to go on the peg." Holding his hand, she guided him through the motion. The ring landed next to the peg.

"Let's try again." She repeated the motion with another ring, successfully circling the peg. "Good job. Let's do it again."

Bill pushed the rings toward her.

She moved the ring toss game aside and handed Bill a large yellow ball. "Let's play catch."

She squatted in front of him. "Bill. Throw the ball here." They volleyed the ball back and forth a few times. "Good job!"

"Let's try the ring toss again." She put the ball aside and set a larger ring toss game in front of him.

He shoved the rings away.

Barb looked at me. "I'm sorry Bill isn't responding to me."

"I wish he would snap to," I said. "He's acting stubborn."

"It's because of the injury." She looked at me sadly. "I'm so sorry to see him like this. I knew him before his accident."

"You did?"

"Yes, he taught on counseling at Lay Ministry Training School when I was a student there."

"What a small world!" I relaxed a bit, reassured by her genuine concern.

"He was a wonderful teacher. I learned so much."

"He really enjoyed teaching that." Bill loved helping people find answers to life's perplexities whether counseling or teaching others what he had learned. Where was my favorite counselor now?

Bill stared into space. Then he tried to get up.

She tried the game again but to no avail.

"I wish he would be himself again." I started to cry.

Barb grasped my hand. "I know it's hard. He'll get better, but it takes time. We'll keep doing what we can."

"Please pray for him, too."

"I am." She squeezed my hand and released it.

The next day we gathered for our first family meeting. Mom, Jody, Joel and I squeezed between the wall and chairs to sit at the end of a long white table in a white room. Three women sat with clipboards and pens on the table in front of them. The rehab doctor darted in and sat. "Sorry I'm late."

From the far end of the table, Julie looked around. "It looks like we're almost all here so let's get started. Shelly from speech should arrive shortly. We are here for a family meeting concerning patient William Barr."

After introducing us, she scanned the other faces. "These people will tell you what department they represent and will report on William."

"I'm Jane from physical therapy. Bill is steadily gaining strength and balance." She described his gradual increase of steps in physical rehab downstairs.

"That's good." I was pleased to hear a good report.

Bump on the Road

"You can take him for brief walks in the hall, but ask a staff person to help you."

"Thanks, Jane." Julie turned toward the occupational therapist. "Barb, how's occupational therapy going?"

"I wish I could say he was doing as well in O.T. Occasionally, he will pick up cues but isn't very responsive. He doesn't follow directions most of the time. We'll keep working with him, but there's not much we can do if he doesn't start responding more."

Julie looked up as another woman entered. "Hi, Shelly. Come on in."

"I'm sorry, my schedule got backed up all morning." Shelly sank into a chair and exhaled as she dropped a stack of papers onto the table.

"No problem," said Julie. "Jane and Barb have given their reports. Are you ready with yours?"

"Sure." Shelly took a deep breath as if to change mental gears. "Part of our job in speech pathology is evaluating when a person is ready to take food by mouth. If they do not understand what to do with food, they are in danger of choking."

"When do you think he can start trying?" I asked. Poor guy. I wouldn't like being deprived of food when others around me ate.

"We'll watch for his readiness but can't hurry it," Shelly replied. "Unfortunately, he doesn't make eye contact and doesn't seem to understand what's being said to him. But soon we hope to try soft foods such as yogurt and ice cream."

"He'll like that. Ice cream is one of his favorites."

"Thanks, Shelly." Julie nodded to a woman wearing scrubs. "This is the charge nurse on this shift. What is your perspective on how Mr. Barr is doing?"

"Mr. Barr is a pleasant man but rarely makes eye contact. He occasionally answers 'yes' or 'no' questions but not other ones such as what is his name or where he lives."

My tigress instinct surfaced to defend my mate. "I've seen some improvement. He's talking more now." This was like a bad parent-teacher conference with my son. *Maybe he's tired of being bossed around by so many women.*

The doctor spoke. "Yes, he's improving but we need to see more than we are now." He paused as he seemed to ponder what to say next. "The head trauma was rather severe. The CT scans we did yesterday show that there is still considerable swelling. Those in our program usually show signs of enough progress to be released within four to six weeks."

My breath stopped midway. I couldn't imagine Bill well enough to go home that soon.

"Some need more time. Then we look at alternate forms of care." He apparently had his doubts, too.

"Alternate forms of care. What would that be?" Mom asked.

"There are a number of fine skilled care facilities in the Twin Cities. They would continue therapies but at a slower pace."

At least it wasn't a nursing home. Or was it? *Please Lord, help him get better quickly! Where's the miracle we've been praying for?*

Discouraged, we returned to Bill's room.

Wearing a tee shirt and lounge pants, Bill looked normal. However, his actions indicated otherwise.

"William won't keep his shirt on." The nurse frowned.

"I know." *Can't you figure out something to do about it?* If the staff didn't know what to do, how would I know?

"Maybe we need to put a hospital gown on him and tie it in back." She opened a cupboard up high and took a neatly folded square from the stack.

Together we stuffed Bill's arms into the sleeves and tied the open-back gown in triple knots at both places on his back. Apparently clothes weren't the clue to acting normal.

Bump on the Road

"There. That should help." Putting one hand on his chest and the other on his back, she turned him around. "William, let's sit down for a bit right here." She maneuvered him to the bedside chair. "There you go. Your wife is here for a visit. In a little bit, you can take a nap when you get tired."

He started to stand. I found the photo album I had brought earlier. "Bill, let's look at some family pictures." I spoke with brassy cheerfulness. "You need to sit down."

He sighed in resignation and sat back in the chair. Briefly.

I opened the album in which I had taped name labels. "Here's a picture of Joel and Bridget and Deanna. Can you believe Deanna's already five?"

He pushed the book away. I persisted. "Here's our son Josh and Angie his wife with their kids Zack and Bree." His chin drifted chestward as his eyelids closed.

The nurse peeked in the door. "How're we doing in here? Are you ready for a little nap, William?"

"I think he is." *If only he would sleep soundly and wake up making sense again.*

She helped him navigate back into bed and I stowed the photos back in the drawer.

I gathered my stuff. "Let's head out."

"That's fine," the nurse said. "We'll keep an eye on him. You have a good day."

"Thanks."

As we walked down the hall, Mom said, "He looks pale and sickly, don't you think?"

"Yeah," said Joel. "He looks mad and frustrated too."

"Poor guy must hate having people tell him what to do," said Mom. "That's probably why he doesn't do the games. He probably thinks it's silly."

Rehabilitation

A couple shuffled past, her arm linked with his. I wondered which one was the patient. The man acknowledged me with a nod. "Is your husband a patient here?" he asked.

"Yes. He was thrown from a motorcycle." Tired of people looking aghast, I didn't say where it happened.

"How's his recovery going?" he asked as the woman looked past me at a spot on the wall.

"He's getting better but not very quickly."

"I know what that's like. My wife had a stroke. Her recovery wasn't going very well, so they were going to send her to a nursing home." He looked at her and back at me.

"Then, about a week and a half ago, she turned a corner. They said she can probably go home tomorrow or the next day." She smiled faintly at his words.

"That's encouraging to hear. I keep hoping Bill will snap out of this."

"He will. I hope the best for you." They continued their hall walk slowly.

❧

At the end of February, I returned to work part time. Since I couldn't do anything to hasten Bill's healing, I was grateful for the diversion of my church office job.

Jody resumed her nurse aide job in a nursing home. It wasn't much of a break. I hoped she wouldn't abandon her goal to become a nurse after being around so much human duress.

We staggered our visits throughout the day, rendezvousing nightly about Bill's progress–or lack of.

"Bill has big circles under his eyes." Mom's face wrinkled with concern. "I don't think he's getting enough sleep."

"I wonder if he sleeps at night," said Jody. "He's drowsy all the time but doesn't sleep very long."

Bump on the Road

"That reminds me." Mom perked up as she remembered something. "Apparently, the aide assigned to him last night knows him from church."

"Really, who would that be?" I tried to remember who worked in hospitals.

"She wrote a note and left it on his bedside stand. Holly was the name."

"I had forgotten that Holly worked at North Memorial. It's a small world!" God had His people stationed all around, looking after my hubby.

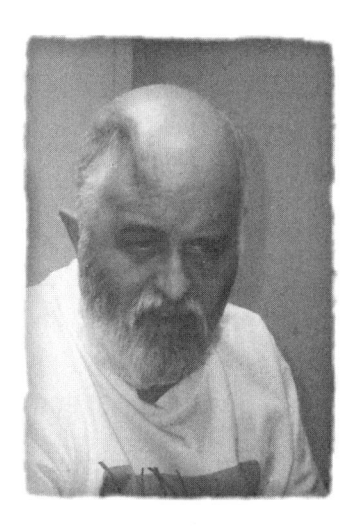

Another Bump

"WHAT SHOULD WE DO about Dad's birthday?" Jody refilled her glass to wash down lasagna and salad.

"That's right, tomorrow is March fourth." Mom shoved her food around her plate.

Peter, our live-in nephew bounded down the stairs, thrusting his arm into a jacket sleeve. "Uncle Bill's birthday is tomorrow? How old will he be?"

"Fifty-three." I sighed. "What a way to spend his birthday!"

Jody finished her water. "I wonder what he'll understand."

"What can we get him?" Mom shook her head. "I'm clueless."

"Maybe we should get a little something now and celebrate later when he's better." Would this be a rerun of Valentine's Day? "He's lost weight from not eating. We could get him a T-shirt and stretchy waist pants."

"I could make a little birthday cake," offered Angie, our daughter-in-law. She and our son Josh had come from Montana.

"Yeah, it might trigger something," said Josh. "Do you think?"

I shrugged. *Something needs to break through the cloud in his brain.*

"Does he like chocolate?" Angie jumped up and headed to the cupboard. "I'll call my mom. She has a recipe for an awesome chocolate cake."

"When should we have it?" asked Mom.

"Let's do it after supper tomorrow. About seven?"

Bump on the Road

"Works for me." Peter looked at the clock. "Bye guys, I'm heading over to the college to work on my paper."

"Now? It's after nine o'clock." Mom shook her head.

"It's okay, Grandma. Three of us are working on a group assignment and it's the only time we can get together."

Jody patted her grandma's hand as Peter dashed out the door.

"He goes a mile a minute." Mom sighed. "Oh, to be young again."

A longing expression lingered on Jody's face. "It feels strange to sit here without homework, but I don't miss the pressure. By the way, I called my advisor at Bethel and found out what classes I need. Bethel doesn't offer them in summer school but my advisor said other schools in the metro have what I need during the summer."

Lord, please help her find the classes and it would be wonderful to see a miracle on Bill's birthday.

The next morning, a nurse called. "I'm really sorry, but I need to tell you what happened."

Oh no, what now?

"We don't know how this happened. It seems that Bill bumped his head during the night."

This is *not* what we wanted for Bill's birthday.

"His left eye was swollen shut and bruised. Today it's still black and blue but not quite as puffy."

"Will he be okay?" *Why hadn't I insisted that they tape a pillow to it like they had done in his other room?*

"We'll take him down for a cat scan this morning and see what's going on in there."

"This won't set him back, will it?"

"I hope not, but there's no way of knowing for sure. I'm so sorry it happened! We'll make sure that someone is attending him all the time. Without the skull bone, his head is not protected."

"Today's his birthday, and I'd hoped he'd have a good day."

"He's sleepy now, and hopefully some rest will help."

"Maybe we should come in a little later today. We wanted to have a small party with family."

"Sounds good. Again, I'm so sorry."

"It's okay. You're doing a good job with him, but could you tape some pillows to the bed rails like they did on fifth floor?"

"I'll see what I can do."

Later that morning, the surgeon called. "The CT scan showed the bruised eye and more swelling of the brain. It will probably take a week or more for the swelling to go down. We'll give Bill a sedative to help him sleep better."

On our way to the hospital, Mom and I bought a T-shirt, knitted lounge pants, and a ball and put them in a yellow gift bag. If nothing else, our grandkids could play with the ball later.

Jody was already there when Mom and I arrived. "Dad looks like he did in India."

Dismally, I agreed. *When will this gravel stretch end and we can get back on pavement?* The dismal journey to recovery was much longer than I had imagined.

"I don't think Dad feels very well. He seems less responsive."

Josh and Angie arrived later. "I kinda threw this cake together. It didn't turn out as well as it usually does."

Josh put his arm around his petite wife. "Looks tasty, Angie."

"Thanks Babe." She smiled adoringly at Josh.

We went to a lounge at the end of the hall. Josh positioned Bill in the middle of the room with his back to the door. We sat around facing him. He stared at the floor without attempting to get up.

Joel and Bridget appeared. "Sorry we're late. Deanna wanted to come but we didn't think it would be good for her to see him yet. Not like this." Bridget set a paper bag on the table. "I brought some paper plates and cups."

Joel glanced at Bill and whispered to me. "He looks terrible." He sat down and shook his head. "Why?" Joel mumbled as he dropped his head into his hands.

We looked at each other's forlorn faces. Attempting to dispel the gloom, Angie said, "Let's sing the birthday song!" Halfheartedly, we sang. No response. So we sang again.

"Bill, it's your birthday." I hoped something would register. "Josh and Angie are here from Montana. Mom, Jody, and I are here. Peter is coming."

"Angie made you a birthday ca..." Josh stopped mid-sentence and looked at me. "Oops. Can he eat it?"

"It's probably not a good idea. Too crumbly," said Jody.

Angie set the cake on the small table behind Josh.

"Dad, here's a gift." Joel put a gift bag on Bill's lap. "It's yours, Dad. Open it." Joel lifted Bill's hand to the tissue. When Joel let go, Bill's hand dropped to his lap.

Joel pulled a shirt from the bag. "Here Dad, we got you this." Joel caught the gift as it slipped through Bill's fingers.

I put another present on Bill's lap. His hands lay limply at his sides. "Here Bill. This is from Mom, Jody and me." Without waiting, I pulled out the contents and gave them to Bill. He handed the ball to Josh. Then he gathered up the shirt and pants and shoved them toward me.

"I think he's tired," said Mom.

I pushed the nurse call button. Once he was wheeled away, we ate birthday cake.

When leaving, we stopped by Bill's room. He surprised me by returning my hug. Perhaps something registered after all.

I shrugged off my coat, mittens, and boots upon returning home the next day. "Welcome home, Sweetie," said Mom. I couldn't see her, but her voice came from the living room. "You must be famished, or have you eaten?" The big green recliner rocked forward as she dislodged herself.

"I had a snack, but I guess I'm sort of hungry."

"Jody's friend brought us another meal." She walked stiffly as though she had been sitting awhile. "It's a yummy meatloaf, cheesy potatoes, and salad. Jody, Peter and I ate some before Peter dashed off to work, but there's plenty left."

"Sounds delicious, but you don't have to wait on me."

"I don't mind. I've been sitting long enough. I fell asleep in the chair and it's too early to go to bed." She opened the fridge and pulled out three foil containers. "Today's mail is over there on the table. You'll be blessed by that one on the top."

Inside a plain white envelope was a folded sheet of lined notebook paper. Emilee Selin, my friend Marilee's daughter, had drawn a detailed scene of Bill lying in a hospital bed. A nurse and doctor stood at his bedside. Angels, twice the size of the people, hovered overhead. Across the top, she had written, "Do not fear. Thine husband shall be healed."

I sat down and cried.

"Isn't that awesome?" Mom set a plate of food in front of me. "How old do you think she is?"

"About seven, I think. This is amazing."

"They're a wonderful family. I'm in awe of Marilee, homeschooling all of those kids." Mom dropped into a chair by me at the table. "Nine kids. Right?"

"Yep. I don't know how she does it."

I had already chosen the Selin family for Jody's future in-laws but hadn't figured out which eligible son would be the best match.

I plowed through the rest of the mail which consisted of health benefit reports, medical bills pending insurance, and get well cards.

Bump on the Road

The next morning, I remained in bed to read my Bible before making an appearance. An Old Testament story caught my eye. The Lord had sent the prophet, Jeremiah, to the potter's house for a message. As Jeremiah watched, the potter smashed a marred pot and reformed the lump of clay. (Jeremiah 18:2-6) I felt as though we were on the potter's wheel, too. The life we had known had been smushed and now the Potter was reshaping us. Apparently, we were a mess if God had to start over.

Reading further in Jeremiah, I pondered God's promise in chapter 29 that He has *good* plans for us. This includes deliverance from our own forms of captivity and exile. If Jeremiah could trust God during bad circumstances, I could too.

Two days after Bill's birthday, we sat with him in rehab's dining room. Mom patted his arm. "How're you feeling today?"

He mumbled in response.

The tall forms of Pastor Gordy and his wife, Jana, appeared in the doorway. "Hi guys!" bubbled Jana. "Here's Bill sitting at the table." She touched his shoulder. "Hi Bill!"

Setting his Bible down, Pastor sat down across from Bill. "Hi Bill. Jana and I came to visit and to pray with you."

Bill reached over and opened Pastor's Bible and started flipping through its pages. Leaving it open, he pushed it aside.

Gordy pulled the Bible toward himself. "This is interesting. Bill opened it to Deuteronomy 20." Pastor read the first portion aloud and patted the open page. "I believe this is a word for you and your family, Bill. God will save you."

Bill acknowledged him with a nod and a quiet "Yes."

"Here's another verse we have been standing on. I think it applies to your situation too." Pastor flipped pages. "This is second Corinthians 1:8-11. It speaks of praying for others in extreme hardships and God's promise of deliverance."

Another Bump

"That fits. Especially the part about trouble in Asia," I said. "It's like a promise from God."

"We're believing God with you." Gordy turned toward Bill. "Yes, Bill, we're praying for total healing."

"Amen." Jana nodded and smiled as she patted Bill's hand.

"Thanks so much for visiting. Your encouragement really helped," I said.

After more conversation and prayer, they left.

Joel, Bridget, and Josh arrived with heavily laden grocery bags.

"Hey Dad, you're looking better today." Josh sat down next to his dad.

"Uh huh." Bill nodded.

"I think so, too," said Mom. She turned toward Bill. "Are you feeling better, Honey?"

Bill nodded.

"We brought supper for you guys." Bridget started pulling containers and baggies of food from the grocery bags. She put it on one end of the table, away from where Bill sat.

Bill looked at Josh. "How are you doing, Josh?"

"I'm good, Dad. How 'bout you?"

Bill mumbled and studied the spread of food.

As fast as he could go, Bill maneuvered his wheelchair to an empty spot by me. After positioning himself at the table, he grabbed a muffin and popped it into his mouth.

"Oh no!" I looked at the others. I shoved the remaining muffins aside. He chewed and swallowed as we watched. When he finished without mishap, our relieved sighs broke the silence in the room.

I dashed out to find Steve, Bill's nurse. "I think Bill's hungry. He just grabbed a muffin and ate it before we could stop him."

"Is he okay?"

"He seems to be. He didn't choke, but do you suppose he could have some ice cream?"

"I'll see what I can do."

Bump on the Road

A few minutes later, Steve came with an ice cream cup and spoon. I peeled back the paper cover and spoon-fed Bill. Though ice cream had been a pre-accident favorite, he didn't relish it as he had the muffin.

Bill turned toward me. "Would you scratch my back?"

I gladly obliged this request, a reminder of our former life.

"His head has more of an indentation now." Joel studied the side of Bill's head where the skull bone had been removed in India. The caving in of his right temple was a sign of progress because it meant that the swelling of the brain was going down. "When are they going to fix that?"

"The doctor said that the swelling needed to go down further and the tissues need to heal." Though Bill wasn't himself yet, I was eager for him to look normal.

"He's better since you sent the email asking for more prayer," Mom said.

"That's true," I replied. "Prayer really works."

I took hold of Bill's hand. "Bill, the Lord is healing you."

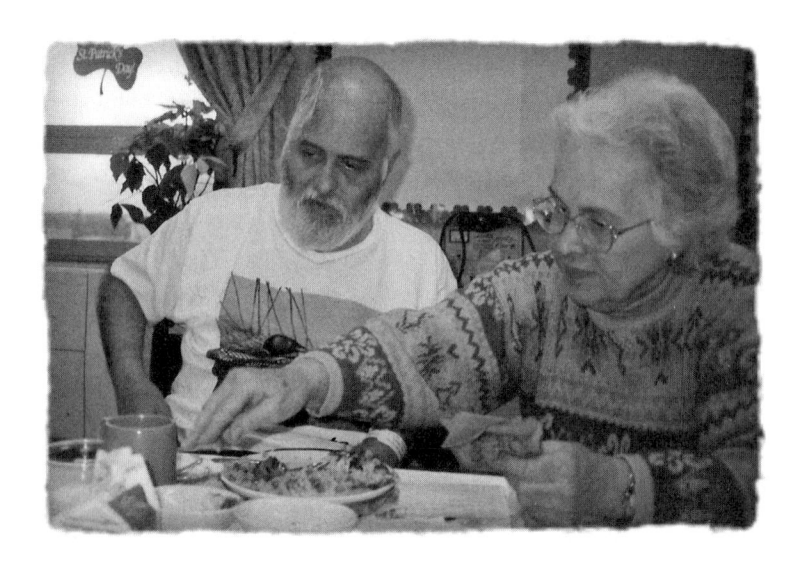

Another Bump

Surgery

MOM AND I sat with Julie at a table in the rehab dining room. Julie folded her hands over the open manila folder lying in front of her. "We had a doctor-therapist-social worker meeting this morning and talked about Bill's situation. The therapists, especially occupational and speech, are only seeing slight improvement. It takes him a very long time to process information."

"I feel like he's getting better," I said. "He seems less agitated and is talking to us more." I wished the therapists could see his little steps as we did. Maybe they simply hadn't found the key.

"That's good," said Julie. "Physically he is getting stronger and is more aware of what's happening around him."

"I wondered if Bill is resistant to all these women telling him what to do." For a man who was used to being independently capable, I couldn't imagine him easily submitting to orders from a changing flow of people.

"I know this is hard," said Julie. "We are doing all we can but, if he doesn't respond to therapy, it doesn't do much good."

"We've wanted to talk to the surgeon after the CT scan yesterday but keep missing him."

"I'm sorry you're frustrated. My role is to be a go-between for families and doctors."

"Don't get me wrong, I appreciate you and your help, but it's frustrating not to talk to the doctor in person. It seems that they could make more of an effort." The Indian doctors talked to us every day, even the surgeon. "Since you're our go-between, can you ask him to please call us at home or talk to us here?"

She nodded. "I'll see what I can do."

In the evening our friend Ron arrived. With one of us on each side of Bill, we walked to a small lounge at the end of the hall. Bill and Ron sat side by side on a couch. I took a chair facing them. Ron described a recent men's retreat. Then he told of his sister who had incurred a brain injury by falling from a horse. She was doing well now. This positive survivor story heartened me.

As Ron's discourse flowed from one topic to another, Bill perked up. When Ron talked about valuing his wife, Bill stood up and hugged me.

Wow. He understood more than I expected.

I urged Ron to come back again and soon. Bill needed some men in his life.

Wednesday morning Bill's neurosurgeon broke the silence by calling before we left home. "The bruising is reducing and swelling has gone down," he said.

"That's good."

"Yes, it is. However, the recent CT scan shows that there is fluid in the ventricles. It's deep in his brain on both sides and in the middle. We see more of this now."

"Why is that? Is it from bumping his head on the bed?" *Oh God, I hope not.*

"Not necessarily. It could be from the accident but is showing up now. Since the swelling has gone down, we can see other things going on. Either fluid was continuing to accumulate or his brain was shrinking and the ventricles were enlarging to fill space."

Why God? Didn't you promise to heal? Bill was serving you. I know You can heal him faster than this.

The doctor continued. "We should be seeing more improvement by now. It's not good to prolong things if it can be

Bump on the Road

avoided." He paused and then continued. "We would like to put in a shunt to drain this extra fluid."

"Will that help him get better?"

"The shunt should increase Bill's chances because it will drain off the excess fluid. It's a mechanical device with a little release valve in it," the doctor replied. "We make a small incision through the back of his head, into his brain, and run it down his neck to drain the fluid into his abdomen where it is absorbed and eliminated. Though I haven't seen it myself, there is a small risk of infection and a slight chance of bleeding. This is true with any surgery."

"What will happen if he doesn't need it anymore? Will it need to be removed?"

"That's usually unnecessary. If there's no fluid to drain, it doesn't do anything. If it quits working and he still needs it, we would operate to replace it. Otherwise, it doesn't hurt anything to leave it there. These shunts usually last about ten years and he probably won't need it at that point, anyway."

For some reason, I felt resistant. "Can we wait a few days to see if he gets better?"

"We'll do another scan in a few days before making a final decision."

Sitting in the rehab dining room that evening, I heard the rattle of the meal cart approaching. Jody glanced toward the door. "I wonder what Dad gets to eat tonight."

"Me too. I hope they got the message that he can have food now." I got up and walked to the doorway to check progress.

Bill sat staring at the table. Jody grabbed his hand. "Dad. You get to eat supper tonight."

"Uh huh."

As he started to push his wheelchair away from the table, an aide entered with a tray. "I have dinner for William Barr."

I felt like celebrating my husband's first meal in six weeks.

She set it before Bill and removed the cover. Three neat hemispheres in varying pastel shades were on a white plastic plate. A small dish held a pale green mound. Another dishful looked like pudding. Then there was a small carton of milk and a brown cup with plastic lid containing coffee. "Enjoy," she said and left.

"Bill, here's your supper. You get to eat." I picked up a spoon and handed it to him.

He studied the spoon and then handed it back to me.

I fed him a bite of the white stuff, then the green stuff. He shook his head as the third item got near. I handed him the spoon. "Here, Bill, can you feed yourself?"

Setting the spoon down, he picked up the milk and sipped some through the straw. Then he took the spoon and returned to the white mound.

"I wonder what all of this is." I read the menu slip. "Mashed potatoes. That would be this white stuff here. He seems to like those. Peas. Must be this green mound. Beef barbecue."

"That must be the pinkish orange stuff." Jody wrinkled her nose and pointed at the remaining mound. "What's this light green stuff?"

"The menu says *tossed salad*." I shook my head. "They wouldn't grind up tossed salad would they?"

Jody discovered a pouch of salad dressing. "Apparently they do."

I tried again. "Bill. You like beef. This is barbecue beef. Why don't you try some?"

He closed his mouth tightly.

"This is pudding, Dad." Jody scooted the vanilla pudding toward Bill. "It's sweet and yummy."

He shook his head and pushed away. Wheeling around the end of the table, he headed for the kitchenette. He reached over and touched the knobs, one at a time. I hopped up and turned his chair away. Never would I have imagined treating my husband as an investigative toddler.

"He's seems to be getting more aware, noticing what's around him," observed Jody.

By supper the next day, Bill had graduated to a *soft mechanical* diet. Quickly he consumed the plateful of cooked carrots, chicken a la king, and canned peaches. Bill had not lost his appetite for real food.

༄

It was Friday morning and I wondered what the day would bring. I took a bowl from the cupboard for my usual—a mixture of granola and flakes. Mom, wearing her bathrobe, sipped coffee. She yawned loudly. "I'm waiting for this coffee to kick in."

The phone rang. It was the neurosurgeon with results from the scan. "Things look the same as they did on Monday, so I think we should pursue the shunt procedure."

I dragged my hand through my uncombed hair and released a heavy sigh. "If it will help him get better, I guess we should go ahead." Rather than wondering *when* Bill would be normal again, I began to wonder *if* he would. It was another overcast day. Like my heart.

"Draining the fluid will probably cause subtle changes. He could get somewhat better over time but he won't recover fully."

God, this is getting increasingly impossible!

That afternoon Mark and Nancy arrived for the weekend. They joined Mom, Jody and me in the rehab dining room for a meeting with the neurologist. A row of scans lined the window sill with outside light showing through the film.

"These are all the scans we've taken since Mr. Barr's arrival," said the doctor. "The spinal fluid in his ventricles is about three times what it should be. This fluid build up is most likely from the accident, not from bumping his head earlier this month."

I hoped he was right. If this was from bumping his head on the bed, I would have had even more *why* questions.

"The shunt should increase chances of further recovery by 50%," said the doctor. "If it works, we'll see improvement right away."

"I guess we should go ahead with it." This seemed to be our only sensible choice.

"Okay. We'll schedule surgery for Monday. When we know the fluid is draining properly, we'll replace the skull piece."

Surely God wouldn't have saved Bill's life for him to be only part of a man. He had committed his life to serving God. Is this what he got in return? Though I had wished Bill would quit wanting to live in India, that sounded better now than this. Much better.

Doctor scanned the faces in the room. His brown eyes showed concern. "Do you have any questions?"

Lots, but none that he can answer.

After the doctor excused himself, I looked around the room at the long faces. They looked as defeated as I felt. Mom grasped my hand. "Are you okay?"

"I guess so."

After the meeting, Nancy followed me to Bill's room. He was awake and tugging on his shirt as though to remove it. I rolled my eyes. Why couldn't he settle down? A change of scenery was usually a temporary fix so I summoned a nurse. She undid the Velcro wrist restraints and helped him into a wheelchair. I pushed him into the lunch room.

A chess game sat on the table. Bill opened the box and studied a black piece briefly before lifting it toward his mouth.

"Bill, don't eat that!" I rescued the knight and pushed the game set out of reach.

"He must think it's chocolate," said Nancy.

Bump on the Road

I returned the chess piece to its box and closed it. "Bill. Let's go for a walk."

Nancy and I guided Bill to standing and went into the hall, one on each side. An older man sat in a wheelchair near the nurses' station as a younger man received discharge instructions. Bill walked up behind, grasped the chair handles and began pushing the man in the chair.

The nurse smiled. "How thoughtful."

We walked slowly alongside as Bill carefully escorted the gentleman down the hall. It was an odd sight – Bill wearing a backwards hospital gown. The man remained stoic.

The young man joined us. "Bill likes to help others," I said.

"Yes, I can see that." He smiled as we approached the elevator. "Thank you for your help," he said to Bill. I will take him now."

Bill paused and then released the handles.

In spite of the chaos in his mind, the Bill who thrived on taking care of people was beginning to emerge.

ഌ

Monday, March 15, Mom, Jody and I arrived at the hospital at 9:00 a.m. to accompany Bill to the surgical area. Two of us held Bill's hands while three nurses worked on inserting an I.V. port. With that finally accomplished, sedatives coursed through Bill as he rolled away to surgical prep.

"Man, that was horrible!" said Jody as we walked out to the waiting area.

"That's the hardest part about this stage. His restlessness." I sighed heavily. "I sure hope this shunt helps."

Through an incision in the back of Bill's head, the surgeon threaded a shunt down Bill's neck into his abdomen. It was a fairly quick procedure that went well according to the surgeon.

Surgery

By 4:00 p.m. that day, the left side of Bill's head had a deep depression, indicating that the shunt was draining fluid properly. Things were looking up. Soon the bone flap would be replaced, protecting his brain, and my husband would look more like himself.

Two days after the shunt installation, the surgeon called and said that they were ready to close up the skull.

"It will be an acrylic piece formed during surgery. It will be as durable as the original."

"It will be a relief to have that closed up," I said.

"Yes, his brain will be protected. We need a bit of artistic license as it may not be possible to get it totally symmetrical."

Oh Lord, please guide the doctor's hand so Bill looks good. Bill's sparse hair wouldn't conceal much.

ഌ

On Thursday, three days after the shunt surgery, Bill returned to surgery for the bone replacement. He was calmer this time, cooperating with the insertion of the I.V. port. Rebuilding Bill's skull with acrylic was a lengthy process. At last, Bill's brain was being covered. Expecting this to conclude Bill's surgeries, we settled into the designated waiting area for the day.

After the operation, Bill went to ICU. Wearing a snug gauze wrapping, he resembled a turban-wearing Sikh *Sadarji* from India. The surgeon told us that things looked good from his surgery in India and that the covering of cranial fluid was still intact.

The next morning, we sat in a small conference room with medical staff and the hospital chaplain for another family meeting.

"Once Mr. Barr is medically stable again, we hope to return him to the rehab floor and therapy," said Bill's doctor. "He needs to make sufficient progress to remain in the program though. If the shunt helps, he'll improve within the next week or two. However, if we don't see enough change, we'll need to arrange for him to go to a skilled care facility."

"I hope he can stay here. We like your program."

"We hope he can, too, but we can't make any promises. At this point, he is generally non-communicative."

"He's been talking to us more," I said.

"Yes, but his behavior is mostly self-directed, not in response to requests that are made of him. He utters phrases but they aren't necessarily related to environmental cues."

I nodded. *Surely our prayers would be answered now. Bill will do so well that they won't kick him out.*

"Mr. Barr has progressed physically but doesn't participate in activities of daily living and remains incontinent. He requires structured supervision and is at risk if left unsupervised." The doctor paused. "I will be gone for a couple of weeks but my partner will fill in. We'll see how things go during that time."

As the meeting adjourned, a nurse came in and handed a note to the doctor. He frowned and shook his head. "This isn't good. Your husband lost movement in his left side, so they ordered another CT scan immediately."

Oh no.

"The scan shows fluid collecting between the cranial piece and the outer layer of his brain. It's pushing the brain over."

I leaned closer to hear him over the sound of my thumping heart. Was it going to drop from seventh floor where I sat all the way to the basement?

"With your consent, they will reopen and attempt to repair whatever is wrong."

"Yes, do what you need to do."

The meeting adjourned and I signed another batch of medical release forms. When we thought Bill was gaining ground, he's going back to surgery. *Lord. Please fix it this time!*

Surgery

Again we headed off to the surgical waiting area. Bill underwent his third surgery in five days. Afterwards, the surgeon described the procedure. "There was a tear, apparently from yesterday's surgery. It was in the outer of three layers around the brain. It was mostly spinal fluid rather than blood."

I nodded and he continued. "We repaired it, inserting two temporary drains and then put the acrylic piece back on."

Before returning home that evening, I stopped by ICU. Bill opened his eyes, said something I didn't understand and moved his limbs. The rehab neurologist entered. "Mr. Barr seems more alert than he was before."

Through the weekend, things seemed stable.

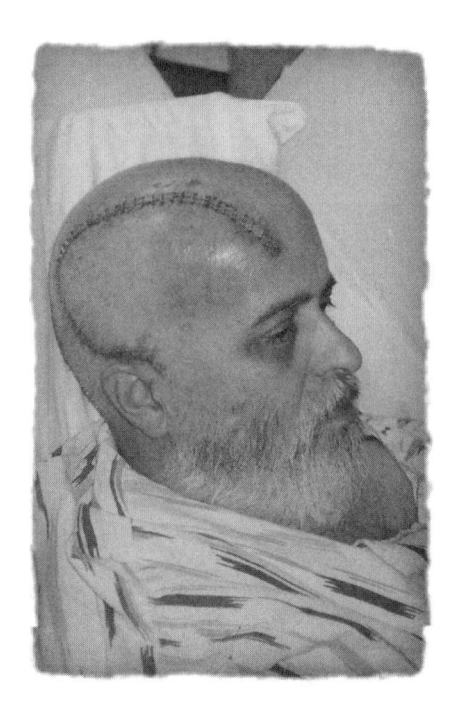

Moving On

EARLY MONDAY MORNING, the surgeon called. "Something still isn't right. William's left side is paralyzed. Fluid is accumulating again where it had been on Friday."

Lord? Where are you?

"Thinking he was mending, we removed the temporary drain tube yesterday. I have not seen this before but I think Mr. Barr needs a permanent way to drain the fluid. We can try a Y on the shunt to drain this area."

"Why is this happening?" I asked.

"It could either be from the original injury or maybe it's just how he's made. We'll operate at 10:00 this morning."

For the fourth time in eight days, Bill underwent surgery. I didn't think I could take any more discouragement. Would they find and fix the problem?

A long morning later, the surgeon appeared. "I believe the procedure was successful," he said. "We'll keep him in ICU and watch him closely."

By the next day, Bill seemed more alert.

Lord, please let this work!

Because he didn't pass his swallowing test, Bill didn't get a meal tray. I watched a nurse unhook the Velcro on the eight inch wide band around his abdomen. She opened a small can of pureed brown food and fed it to Bill through his stomach tube.

"I'm curious. What kind of food does he get that way?"

She turned the can around and read the ingredients. "It has beef, peas, green beans, peaches, orange juice, canola oil and a full array of vitamins and minerals."

Two days later, on Wednesday, Bill graduated from ICU to the neurology floor. Soon he would return to rehab.

☙

"Let's go to the chapel. There's more room there." Mom's friend Pat apparently felt as crowded in Bill's quarters as I did. Bill was in an unknown region of his mind, so Mom, Jody and I followed Pat downstairs. Usually we hurried past the room labeled CHAPEL. Maybe it was because I had associated it with bereavement. Now I wondered if death would have been easier. Guilt crept over me like a blanket on a hot muggy day. *I should be grateful he's alive.*

Light filtered through stained glass depicting Jesus in the Garden of Gethsemane. We sat in a cushioned pew in the center. I was glad no one else was there.

Pat brightened. "Remember the three women who went to the garden tomb, expecting to anoint Jesus' body for burial?" she whispered. "But He wasn't there. He had been resurrected. You three women. You're like those three. Keep praying and believe for Bill's resurrection. The same God who raised Jesus from the dead can bring Bill back."

Easter was coming. Would we have our own resurrection miracle?

By Thursday Bill's condition had stabilized. Yet, I felt defeated. The long haul was pressing in. Julie said that they hadn't taken Bill back to the rehab floor and that the doctor wanted us to find another facility for him.

In the privacy of the brown velvet seated Olds, I talked to God about how I missed my husband – the Bill that was typically "there" for us, the Bill who made people his first priority, the doting spouse Bill. Whenever things went wrong, he was there to hug and console me. Now I needed consolation *because* of him. *Lord, I read in the Bible that you are a husband to widows. I sure feel like a widow right now. Please be my husband.*

I thought about the bounty of finances and prayer pouring in from around the globe. This was God's love through people. Our email list continued growing. Even people whom I had not met were praying for us. Occasionally, we received cards from someone we hadn't seen for many years. The most surprising one was from a pastor with whom Bill had worked as a mere seminary student thirty years earlier. Apparently Bill's accident had been included in the College of Wooster alumni newsletter that I had ignored. The ever expanding network of concern strengthened me as I traversed the deepest valley I had ever known.

Back home, I sat at the table eating another late supper.

"How was Bill tonight?" Mom looked up at me as she scrubbed a pan in the kitchen sink.

"I think he's better. He was more alert. He even asked to use the bathroom." I took another bite of baked chicken. "He kept pulling his gauze turban off. After the third time, the nurse said it was okay to leave it off."

"It's probably getting itchy." She rinsed the pan and set it in the drain basket. "How does his incision look?"

"He has a zillion half inch staples all along here." I ran my finger from above my right eyebrow up over my head and down to the top of my ear. "It's indented where they made the incision."

I tried not to think about my disappointment when I saw Bill's uncovered head. The top of his ear stuck out and there was an indentation above his ear. The doctor was right. Surgeons are not artists. I wished Bill had more hair.

Jody came downstairs and joined me at the table.

"How's it going, daughter dear?"

"Okay, I guess. I was trying to figure out summer school but couldn't concentrate." She sighed heavily. "I feel badly because I think I left Dad in India on bad terms."

"Really? I don't remember that," I said.

"He was trying to help us with all the arrangements for traveling and I was annoyed that he didn't think we could do it on our own. I guess I was trying to prove to myself that I was a grown up. I was really rude."

"I don't think it was that bad."

"I long to make it right, to show him the respect that he deserves. I wish I could thank him for watching out for us. Now I realize how much I need and want his advice."

I put my arm around her and held her as she cried. "Lord, you know Jody's heart and You forgive us for these things. If she needs to make this right with her dad, we trust You to make it possible." I doubted that he thought about it now.

Deliberately changing to a positive note, I said, "Tonight Bill turned his wheelchair toward a stack of magazines. He picked them up one at a time and started flipping through the pages. Occasionally he licked his finger to grab and turn a page.

"I can picture him doing that," said Mom.

Though minute, this felt like progress.

"Have you gotten to talk to that elusive rehab doc yet?"

"Nope. I'm so frustrated. He's always gone by the time we get there and he hasn't bothered to call."

Mom slapped the counter. "That's not right. The least he could do is talk to you on the phone, don't you think?"

"I feel like we're pawns in the hands of a doctor who doesn't care. I sure hope the regular doctor comes back soon. He had said that Bill could try the rehab floor after surgery but it doesn't seem like this doctor is going to let that happen."

"The poor guy had four surgeries in eight days." Mom grabbed the towel hanging from the oven door and vigorously dried her hands. "No wonder he's moving slowly. He needs time to rest and heal."

"I agree. Let's hope they see it that way, too."

෮ඏ

Sunday after church we entered Bill's room to see friends Ray and Sue smiling broadly. They reported that Bill had been sleeping when they arrived, but then he opened his eyes and greeted them by name. I was amazed that he recognized them *and* remembered their names.

When another couple arrived later, I hoped for a repeat performance. He quietly said "Hi" and closed his eyes for another nap.

Five weeks had passed since our return from India. Perhaps Bill would improve now if given a chance.

The next day, a petite woman sat by Bill's bed. She leaned toward him and said, "I'm Lori, from speech pathology. We're going to play a game. Okay?"

She drew a grid and handed the paper to him. "Bill, let's play tic tac toe." She made an "X" and gave the pencil to Bill. He held it a second but returned it to her. She tried again but elicted the same response.

She patted his arm. "I'm going to ask you some questions."

Continuing to stare blankly at the floor, Bill mumbled or remained silent in response. She handed him a yellow pad. He took the pencil, wrote, and returned the pad to her.

She studied it, shook her head and handed the paper to me. "Can you tell what he's written?" Though the squiggly lines resembled Bill's writing, it wasn't legible.

She held a spoonful of pudding to his lips. He opened his mouth to receive the food and worked it around, clearing his throat frequently.

"I'm concerned that he's not swallowing adequately because he clears his throat often." She asked him more questions but he responded like a statue.

"If I could get him to talk, I could evaluate the clarity of his voice." She patted his hand and tried another time. "That's another way of testing his readiness to swallow."

I felt like shaking him and yelling "TALK TO HER!" If only he would babble to her as much as he did to us.

"I'm sorry. I don't think he's ready but we'll try again tomorrow."

Later, his occupational therapist saw the paper and was surprised to learn that Bill had written it. She had tried unsuccessfully to get him to hold a pen. She left a tablet and pen in case he got inspired to write more.

Another CT scan was done March 30. The tubes now functioned properly, draining excess fluid. Since the swelling had diminished, more bruising could be seen. The doctor said that this indicated significant deficits.

Help Lord! We need your resurrection power! I identified with the woman in Luke 18 who continuously hounded the unrighteous judge until he finally paid attention. I also felt like I was being run over by one of the noisy diesel trucks in India. Why would God save Bill's life but leave him incomplete? His life has a *purpose*. Not *this*. Again, I wondered if death would have been easier. I shuddered. *Help, Lord!*

As Joel had said a few days earlier, "God, you made him. You can fix him!"

Desperate

MOM, JODY AND I went to the hospital extra early the first day of April. Before going to Bill's room, we stopped at the nurses station and told them we needed to meet with the doctor. Good news—he was still on the premises. The nurse told us to wait in the family lounge.

A little while later, a stocky, middle-aged doctor entered and introduced himself. My anger dissipated as I sat across from an actual human being.

I told him I was concerned about Bill adjusting to a new place as he was starting to get back on track after a series of surgeries. He listened patiently, then explained that the rehab unit was for those who showed enough progress to return home after six to eight weeks. Six weeks had passed since Bill was admitted into the rehab program. I couldn't imagine Bill going home in two weeks. Insurance could suddenly stop payment and we would be left with a frightful bill.

The doctor said that insurance would provide coverage longer in a skilled care facility. Bill would have therapies at a less demanding pace.

"Our primary concern is his language, memory, and decision-making or judgment skills. You may see 80%, 60%, or 20% recovery. We have never seen 100% recovery. There's no way of knowing how much he will improve. He'll reach plateaus and stay there awhile. At some point, he'll level off and remain there. Only time will tell."

Why wouldn't Bill shake loose and start paying attention? At times I felt like giving up and going on with my life as though he didn't exist.

"What is a skilled care facility? Is it ... a nursing home?" I asked.

"They're often called that but many younger people in your husband's situation receive care there and do well. Julie will help you find a place."

"Thank you very much for meeting with us, Doctor." I felt better about this neurologist now that we had finally conversed with him.

Early afternoon, Julie gave us information about several options and encouraged us to look at the facilities before visiting Bill the next day. "Just go drop in. You don't need to make an appointment. That way you see them in action without their trying to make a good impression. See what would be a good fit."

Unless things changed drastically, Bill wasn't going back to the rehab floor. Our only choice was to trust God to take care of Bill, preparing the right place for his next stage of recovery. Certainly, God would not abandon him. His life was spared. If Bill's purpose on earth was finished, he wouldn't have lived through this. I needed to leave the details and Bill's recovery in God's hands. Only He could solve this problem.

Mom and I went upstairs to rehab to collect Bill's belongings. This felt like another step backwards, more dashed hopes. Many of the staff had become friends, not only caring for Bill but also for us. I remembered the nurse who had assured us that she was praying for Bill. When Bill had a particularly rough day, an aide had hugged and talked to Jody for a long time.

The head nurse helped gather Bill's things. As she held open a large plastic bag for me to fill, I wept. "You have been so good to him," I said. "I wish he didn't have to leave here."

Bump on the Road

She smiled sadly. "Don't give up. Some need more time to heal. He'll keep getting better. We often have former patients come back after going to a nursing home. We're amazed by how well they're doing."

Loaded up with two bags each, Mom and I trudged back to Bill's room on the neurology floor.

It was the Thursday before Easter. Putting my husband in a nursing home hardly seemed like God's best plan. Why wouldn't the doctor change his mind and start counting weeks from now? Bill was finally getting better. Clearly he had asked, "Please get water in both of these cups" as he handed two Styrofoam cups to me.

That afternoon, Mom, Jody, Joel and I circled our city in search of Bill's next home. This felt wrong. Terribly wrong. A nursing home for *my* husband with his *mother* helping. At age 53, Bill was too young to sit around with old folks. I felt sick. Would we finish our marriage with him in a nursing home?

I had unpleasant memories of visiting such places. Again, I was being stretched outside of my comfort zone.

We toured four places that day where we saw sad people Mom's age and older. Some moved slowly with walkers. Others sat in chairs. A few greeted us, but most were sullen.

We talked with nurses and therapists, wanting to make sure Bill would receive continued help and attention. When we returned to the hospital with the results of our exploration, we felt better. Maybe this was for the best, after all. Our first choice was at a lovely lakeside setting with a pleasant interior. Another place appealed to us because of its separate area for younger people.

Julie faxed Bill's medical reports to these facilities so they could evaluate whether they could take him. We had good options, or so we thought.

Friday morning, questions cut my sleep short. The ratio of staff to patients would be lower. Would Bill get suitable help when he needed it? Would he hurt himself again because someone wasn't watching him all the time? Hope waned like last night's moon.

I ruffled through my closet absently, reminding myself to keep trusting God. He had spared my husband's life. He could take care of him now, too. I put on the same clothes I had worn the day before. The morning was quickly disappearing and I had lots to do before I could leave the house.

An overdue bill for Bill's flight sat on the kitchen table. Back in India, East West Rescue had agreed to let us send the payment for Bill's flight after we got home. I thought the insurance company had promised payment within seven days. I called the helpful insurance agent who had managed Bill's case earlier. After going through several menu items and waiting on hold, I found out that she was no longer responsible for our case. I panicked.

Our new agent said that the check had been cut ten days earlier. Apparently, it was stuck somewhere between their office and our house. Anxiety mounted. I didn't have time to track down a lost check. I pled with the woman to look into it. She connected me to someone else who said that they wouldn't put a tracer on it unless it had been over two weeks since the check was issued. I halfheartedly thanked her and hung up. I hoped she was right.

The Bible said that God made a *helpmate* for Adam. Now this meant my being Bill's advocate. As the youngest in my family, I was accustomed to deferring to others and being taken care of. I had carried this attitude into marriage. Now I was the caretaker. At age 51, I was finally growing up. Bill used to handle the complicated paperwork. Now it was up to me. Though Mom and Jody wanted to help, they couldn't do what I hated doing the most. I had to persist when I felt like stopping. I had to shake off passivity and become a fighter.

Bump on the Road

God is greater than any problem I have. Yes, Lord, forgive me for forgetting that!

My part was to trust God and lean on Him like never before. This was a day by day choice. In spite of his despair, Job believed in God and said, "I know that you can do all things; no plan of yours can be thwarted." In the end, Job's situation turned for the better. I would keep believing for that, too.

During the first weeks after the accident, I was in a numb stupor and could drift with the process. Now I had to fight for Bill's welfare. I couldn't be passive or give up.

I remembered the conversation with Pat in the chapel. After making a second cup of tea, I reflected on that day's devotional reading. *Lord, you made the heavens and the earth. Nothing is too hard for you.*

With man this is impossible, but with God all things are possible. Would Easter bring resurrection of Bill – all the way?

൧

Easter dawned with me dubiously hopeful. Attending church preceded the daily hospital trek. We had communion during which I realized that I had taken Bill for granted until now. What had seemed important previously paled now in contrast. Perhaps I needed to surrender more fully to God and be more passionate about serving Him. Did my apathy cause Bill's accident? Did God allow this because I was so self-centered?

O God, I'm sorry. Please forgive me. Tears streamed down my face as I rummaged in my purse for a tissue.

A gentle inner voice assured me that God works all things together for good.

We left church, loaded. Members of an extended family had made extra for their family celebration so they could share with us. Buoyed by their love, we went to the hospital.

Desperate

"Happy Easter!" Bill's Puerto Rican roommate, Angel, greeted us. He raised his bed to sitting position.

"Happy Easter to you, too."

Bill watched as I set a grocery bag on his table.

"I am praying for your husband to be healed," said the little elderly man.

"Thank you so much." My eyes moistened. "We will pray for you, too."

"I'll see if we can take Dad down to the cafeteria," said Jody.

Angel sat up and lowered his feet slowly to the floor. Grasping the bed, he edged around it to Bill's side. Clasping hands with us, he prayed. When finished, he shuffled back to bed. Soon he was asleep.

"It's as though there really is an angel in this room," whispered Mom. "I don't remember ever seeing him get out of bed before."

"Me neither." I shook my head. "Lord, bless him."

Pushing a wheelchair, a nurse returned with Jody. "William, your family has brought you Easter dinner. They are going to take you down to the cafeteria to eat." She turned to me. "They aren't serving food down there now so you'll have plenty of space to yourselves."

The nurse assisted Bill into the wheelchair. Then Mom and I followed Jody as she pushed her dad downstairs to the cafeteria.

Jody positioned him at the end of a long table and locked the chair into place. He attempted to move but to no avail.

"Dad, here's Easter dinner. Look at this yummy food."

"Silly chair won't move," said Bill. He fidgeted with the wheels and sighed again.

"Go ahead and get it ready. I'll take him for a spin around the room." As the others set out food, I rolled Bill back and forth between the rows of tables. As long as we kept moving, he remained seated. Then I returned him to his spot at the head of the table.

Bump on the Road

Bill devoured Jell-O, sweet potatoes, cheesy potatoes, rolls, ham, salad, and cake. Then he tried again to excape his chair.

We packed up the leftovers and returned to Bill's room. He chattered about babies, dogs, and a church choir. I wondered if he was recalling when Joel and Jody took him to see the babies on the maternity floor. Perhaps he also remembered the pet therapy dog from earlier in the week and the choir which sang one Sunday for rehab patients.

A nurse attempted to put a thermometer behind Bill's ear. He pushed her hand away so she let him hold it to see what it was. He grasped it as a microphone, held it to his mouth, and began to speak.

Bill was making small steps of improvement but there was no obvious Easter miracle.

The next day was Monday. Time to get serious about finding a new place. Unless.

I'm not giving up hope. Yet.

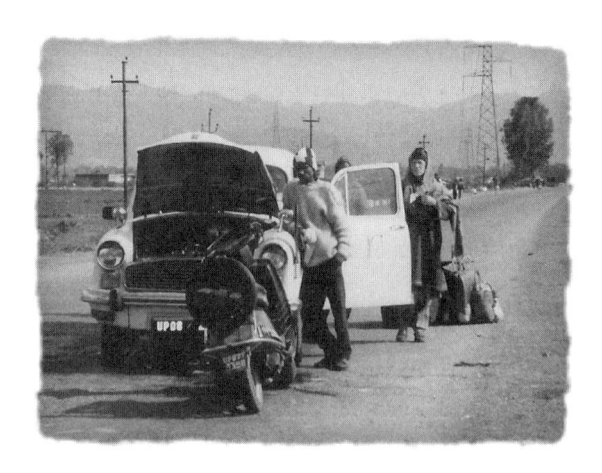

There Must Be a Place

BILL'S NEUROLOGIST returned to work but agreed with the other doctor. Insurance could stop paying suddenly without warning so we had to find an alternative. Now. I felt like a heartless system was pushing us around.

The facilities we had chosen weren't staffed for constant surveillance of my mobile husband. We had to keep looking. Bethesda Hospital was the only option equipped for Bill's needs, but it was the same level of care as North Memorial. Would insurance pay?

Lord, we need a place where Bill can get better! This seems impossible, but nothing is impossible to You.

Bill seemed to know that he was leaving.

On one of our walks in the hall, he approached the nurses' station and said, "I need my shoes."

"You have some in your room." I tugged him back toward his room. "Let's go get yours."

Mom opened his closet and frowned. "I don't see any in here, do you?"

When I didn't see them either, I got down on my knees and looked under both beds. Then I checked his roommate's closet. No shoes. Angel had gone to a nursing home that morning.

Bill and I returned to the nurses' station. "I need my shoes," he said.

"We can't find his anywhere," I added. "We looked all over but they aren't in his room. Do you know where they might be?"

"When Angel's family came to take him to the nursing home, we tried to figure out what things were his. We asked the men, but neither knew."

"Oh no." I laughed nervously. "Some clothes are left in the closet but they aren't Bill's."

"I'm so sorry." She shook her head. She called Angel's nursing home and arranged for Mom to swap Angel's clothes for Bill's shoes.

Bill begged me to remove my loafers. After squeezing his feet into them, he started off for the nurses' station again. "I *need* my shoes."

"She doesn't have them." I redirected Bill back to his room where he pulled off my socks. He took off again, so I followed in my bare feet.

"Bill, they *don't* have your shoes." I took his elbow and rotated him back down the hall. He sighed, shook his head, and obliged.

He sat down next to his bed.

"Bill. I need my socks. Can I have them back?" What happened to my ultra-flexible spouse who was rarely bothered by inconveniences? This was another change from the old Bill.

He laughed humorlessly as he removed and returned my footwear. Then he crawled into bed and went to sleep.

༂

The next morning, a Bethesda representative met us at North Memorial. "We evaluated Bill's situation and have decided that we can try Bill in our rehabilitation program. He needs to continue therapies and improve steadily to remain in our program, though."

"Thank you!" I felt like hugging the woman.

We flew into action, filling several large bags with three months' worth of acquisitions – get well cards, helium balloons, clothing, plants, photo albums, and more. Within an hour, two medics belted Bill into a wheelchair and escorted him to a medical transport vehicle outside.

Mom paused as she stuffed shirts into a bag. "Another chapter. I wonder how he'll do."

"Me too. It's his first time outside in three months."

"Do you think he understands what's happening?" She sat on the empty bed.

"I don't know. Sure hope he adjusts okay." I grabbed a bag to fill.

"Poor guy is being bounced from pillar to post." Mom sighed heavily and rose slowly.

"That's for sure." I removed several pictures taped to the brick wall. "With all this stuff, it's a good thing we have both of our cars here."

We finished gathering Bill's accumulation. A nurse brought in a cart and helped us haul everything downstairs. She waited as Mom and I fetched our cars from the parking ramp to load.

I led the way through Minneapolis to downtown St. Paul, getting us lost once. We found our way out and drove through rush hour traffic to Bethesda, located in the shadow of the state capitol.

After parking in a ramp, we grabbed some bags and rode an elevator to fourth floor. The door opened to a nursing station.

"We're here to see my husband, Bill Barr," I said to the women behind the desk. "He was brought here a little while ago."

She looked at a list and then shook her head. "Is he on the locked unit?"

"Yes, I think so."

She pointed to a secured area. "Ring the buzzer over there by the double doors. Someone will help you shortly."

Peering through the window, I saw people walking around inside. Finally, a nurse opened the door partway.

"I am Bill Barr's wife and this is his mom. He was brought here from North Memorial a little while ago," I explained.

Bump on the Road

"Come in. I'll take you to his room."

We followed her through a large, round room. A man strolled past wearing a helmet that covered most of his head. An abrasive female voice came from the TV area. Others sat in chairs around the room. Most were expressionless.

A young man popped into my personal space and greeted me loudly. I was relieved that an employee immediately apprehended him and gently reminded him to leave visitors alone.

This was the "behavior modification unit." Patient rooms were located around the circumference of the large central area. The staff person invited us to sit in Bill's room, saying that Bill's nurse would be in shortly. She left, closing the door behind her.

I sighed in relief. It was hard enough to face Bill like this, let alone strangers. I missed my soul mate, the man that Bill had been. Now his brain took me into a realm I didn't understand. The fragile thread of normalcy had broken, trading reality for illusion.

Bill lay with cloth bands strapping his wrists to the side of the bed, snoring quietly. The large pie shaped room had a large window, built-in shelves, a small closet, and a bathroom adjoining. There was plenty of space for his collection of memorabilia as well as the two huge drawings from a church friend. Using markers on large sheets of brown wrapping paper, she had drawn declarations of faith in Jesus for Bill's healing. I wondered when he would notice the expressions of love surrounding him.

"Go ahead and sit, Mom." I motioned to the lone chair.

"What about you? You're tired, too, aren't you?"

"This is fine." I perched on the wide window ledge, envisioning it filled with cards.

A tall African man entered. "Hello. I'm Mo, Bill's nurse tonight." He shook our hands and we introduced ourselves.

He pulled two chairs in from the main room and closed the door. "Please have a seat. We need to do some paperwork." Mo handed me a clipboard with forms. "Tell me about your husband and what happened."

After hearing my story and completing the admissions paperwork, Mo affirmed Bethesda's ability to help and left.

"I like him, don't you?" Mom asked.

"Yes, I do. This is going to be okay."

A few minutes later, a knock on the door preceded a tall, slender man with slightly graying hair. "Hello, I am Dr. Rupp," he greeted. "I'm here to do a brief intake exam on Mr. Barr."

As the doctor checked Bill's vitals, Mom asked, "By any chance, have you worked at a hospital in Africa?"

"Yes, I have," he replied, giving the hospital name.

"Do you know Bruce and Kathy?" Mom asked. "He's a doctor and she's a nurse. They've spoken highly of a Dr. Rupp."

"Yes, I certainly do!" He broke into a large smile. "We worked together. They are fine people."

"They're good friends of ours. Small world!"

I remembered something else. "Do you have a daughter, Jody, who attended Northside for a year?"

"I do!" he replied.

"Our daughter, Jody, and your Jody were friends in fifth grade."

"That's right, I remember your Jody coming to our house," he said.

"This is so cool," said Mom. "Isn't God good?"

"I'm sorry we meet under these circumstances." Dr. Rupp wrinkled his brow with concern. "Would it be all right if I pray with you before I leave?"

"Yes, please do."

He prayed for natural and supernatural healing for Bill and for God's peace to be in our hearts. Meeting him that first night at Bethesda felt like confirmation of God's care. He really was looking after Bill. And us.

Bethesda

AT ELEVEN O'CLOCK the next day, I stood outside the locked double doors waiting. Peering through the window, I recognized the gregarious man from the night before. He walked toward the door but a staff woman redirected him. Then she came and cracked open the door. "Can I help you?"

"Yes, I'm here to visit Bill Barr, my husband."

She hesitated before motioning for me to enter. "Visiting hours are only in the evening, from six until eight." She made sure the door locked securely behind us.

"One of the nurses last night told us that family could come during the day, too."

She shook her head. "It must have been the new employee. We keep our patients busy during the day with therapies and other activities so we need to limit visiting hours. On Saturdays and Sundays visiting hours are from noon until eight."

I was used to North Memorial where they invited visitors anytime throughout the day. "Since I live a half hour away, may I see him now since I'm already here?"

"Yes, come on in." She led me to his room. "He hasn't begun therapies yet. A doctor will evaluate your husband this morning. Then he'll start."

"Thank you." I slipped into Bill's room, feeling like a dog that had sneaked onto the forbidden couch. Bill sat in a vinyl covered recliner with wheels. Cloth restraints held him in place.

Soon a tall man in white overshirt arrived. "Good morning." He extended his hand in greeting. "I'm one of the neurologists here. Are you Mrs. Barr, William's wife?"

"Yes, I am." I shifted to the opposite foot. "I hope I'm not in the way."

"Absolutely not. I'm going to do an evaluation. You may observe if you would like." After introducing himself to Bill, the doctor pushed Bill, chair and all, around the corner to a table in the main area. He sat facing Bill while I sat to one side. "William. Or do you go by Bill?"

Bill nodded.

"We call him Bill," I was getting used to talking for my formerly talkative spouse.

The doctor asked Bill if he knew where he was, what happened to him, and what year it was. My husband remained stone-faced and silent.

"I'm sorry he's not talking to you. He hasn't always been this way."

The doctor glanced down at the papers in front of him. "January 26. It's been about two and a half months." He adjusted his glasses. "This is still fairly early in the recovery process. He seems to be moving along fairly normally."

Relief welled within. "That's encouraging. Thanks for letting me sit in on this."

"No problem at all." He patted Bill's hand and said, "We'll get you better so you can get out of here. Okay, Chap?"

Bill nodded.

The doctor wrote notes on the paper and said, "We'll try again after he's settled in a bit." turning to Bill, he said, "I'll see you again." Patting Bill's shoulder, he stood and handed some papers to a nurse who stood at my eye level when I was seated. Our niece Joy wasn't the only shortie around.

Bump on the Road

As the neurologist strode away, the nurse stayed. "Your husband will get better. This is a good place for him. We had one man who was much worse than this when he came. Now he's back at his job. His wife said he's even happier than he used to be."

"That's encouraging to hear." I wiped my eyes and fumbled for a tissue.

"It was unusual because patients usually battle depression. We're aware of those issues and help as much as we can."

"I hadn't realized we weren't supposed to come this early so I'll come during visiting hours from now on," I said.

"Don't worry about it,"the nurse answered.

"Thanks. I was wondering something, though. Our daughter is going into nursing and works evenings in a nursing home. She wants to see her dad but can't always get here during visiting hours. Can she come during the day when Bill's not busy with therapy?" I wanted to ask if I could observe therapy, but didn't want to push my luck.

"I don't see why not but I'll check with my supervisor."

I left that morning with mixed emotions tumbling about. Whereas the environment was less hectic, I felt depressed. I wondered if it was because of seeing a cluster of lives altered by head injury or if there was some sort of depressive spirit there. I hoped that he would make enough progress to move into a less restricted area. Maybe that would help. Though this was a hospital, it felt like an institution. I remembered a miserable summer during college when I worked at a state institution for the mentally retarded. After one girl had yanked my hair, I resolved to avoid such places.

When Mom and I visited the next day, the tall African man was Bill's nurse again. Suspecting that Bill was tired of being bossed around by women, I hoped that Bill would respond well to Mo's gentle authority. "How's Bill doing today?" I asked.

"He seems to be adjusting. He's eating well, drinking water, and slept about five hours last night once he settled down about 2:30. He seemed anxious, though."

Bill turned his head toward us when he realized we were there. "Hi Mom. How are you?"

Mom beamed. "I'm good, Honey. How are you?"

Bill stood and we followed him into the common area. He patted the large purse that was hanging from Mom's arm. "Do you have something for a headache?"

She dug in her purse. "No, I can't find anything."

"I'll go ask the nurse," I said. Mo was busy so I talked to a nurse at the desk. She checked Bill's chart and gave him liquid pain reliever.

Even so, Bill continued asking for pain medicine. He spotted a small piece of white paper on the floor and reached for it. Before he got it to his mouth, I grabbed his arm. "No, Bill. That's dirty. The nurse gave you Tylenol."

"Do you have anything for my headache in your purse?" he repeated. He wasn't giving up.

I faked a purse search. "No. The nurse gave you some. You'll feel better soon." I patted his forearm. "Wait a little longer."

We followed him back to his room where he slipped my purse off my shoulder and looked in the top layer of contents. "I need the keys." He searched through his clothes hanging in the closet. "I need an address." Then he poked around in my coat pockets.

Perseveration. We had learned this word at North Memorial. A common result of brain injury, perseveration describes being stuck on one thought or idea. Bill's new pattern was to lock into something and not let go until he slept off the notion in exchange for another. *Oh Lord. How long will this last?*

Bill's brain resembled scrambled eggs. He seemed desperate to make sense of his strange surroundings and life. The literature from North Memorial recommended familiar, orderly environ-

Bump on the Road

ments. His life was anything but that. He had spent the past two and a half months in unnatural places with strangers caring for him. At least this room wasn't cluttered.

Home was a different story. Bill's makeshift basement workshop was in disarray because he had barely finished a project before we left for India. The aftermath was left for cleaning up later. I hoped we could figure out what to do with the tools and scraps of wood spread throughout our basement before reintroducing him to home.

ಸಿ

"Why did we even bother driving all the way down here?" I said to Mom as we followed Bill across the large central room. "He acts like he's avoiding us."

She nodded her head understandingly. When Bill eased into a chair in front of the T.V., Mom and I sat on straight back chairs on the periphery.

Turning toward me, a woman huskily declared, "I'm so sick of this place. They told me I could go home but I'm still here."

"How long have you been here?" I asked.

"Since last summer." She fussed with her leg brace. "Hey you. Nurse," she yelled. "Take me back to my room, would ya?"

"Hi yah." It was the same extroverted young man. "How'r you?" He waved in my face.

I turned toward Bill as if he would rescue me. Instead, he rose and ambled toward his room. I looked at Mom who was listening to a patient's quiet rambling. She nodded occasionally. Then Mom patted the man on his hand and excused herself. *Oh Lord, if only I were as patient as Mom.*

Back in his room, Bill jiggled the bathroom door handle. "Humph. They keep locking me out."

I intercepted a nurse and asked her to let him into the bathroom.

"We keep it locked because patients flush things down. Like underwear and socks. Earlier today his toilet was plugged so we had to call maintenance." She unlocked the door, let Bill in and stood guard outside, with her ear close.

The toilet flushed and Bill started to come out.

"Did you wash your hands?" She pointed toward the sink.

He turned around and did as reminded. Then he walked out and sat in the recliner in his room.

The nurse leaned toward me and spoke quietly. "He keeps using the bathroom every few minutes. I can't imagine he really needs to go that often. That's why we keep an eye on him."

"Uh huh." I had also noticed his frequent trips.

"Bill, let's look at some pictures." I picked up a photo album. "Here are some pictures of our family." I sat next to him and opened the book to a picture of our granddaughter sitting on his lap.

He pushed it aside, stood and walked away.

"This is so frustrating!" I smacked the album onto the table. "It's as though he doesn't even care if we're here."

Mom took my hand. "I know. It must break your heart."

I nodded and sniffled. "This is so unlike how Bill used to be."

"I know. I'm so sorry."

I laughed dryly. "It's not your fault."

"Maybe if I weren't here, he would pay more attention to you."

I shook my head vehemently. "I doubt it. Besides, I want you here. I need your moral support."

"I hope I'm that, at least."

"You are. Absolutely." I pulled her into a hug and we cried together.

Then I looked up to the welcome sight of Phil and Janie, our friends who had played music at North Memorial. Phil carried a familiar long black case. Their coming was a drink of fresh water in a desert. "It's so good to see you!"

Bump on the Road

"It's good to be here," said Janie. "The nurse said that Phil can set up his keyboard in the adjacent conference room so that we can have privacy and not disturb the others."

"Bill, Phil and Janie are here. He brought his keyboard. Let's go into this room over here." He looked at me blankly so I grabbed his hand. "Come on Bill. We're going over here with Phil and Janie." He rose as reluctantly as a teenage boy to do chores. I pulled him across the common room. At the doorway he hesitated, mumbled something and tried to pull his hand from my grasp. A nurse coaxed him from the other side and he walked into the room and sat down.

Phil set up his keyboard on the long table and began to play. Bill stood and walked to a closed door.

"There's a choir in here," he said. "I need to go in."

"Bill, don't you want to stay here and listen to Phil's music? He came to play for you."

"Someone needs to help me. I must go in there." Then he reached toward the door back into the common area.

I looked at the nurse, expecting her to somehow influence him. Instead she opened the door and followed him out to where he sat by other patients in front of the TV.

Turning toward Janie, I said, "You came all this way and he walks out on you. I'm sorry."

She embraced me. "It's okay, Cheryl."

I sobbed in her arms. "I thought he would relax and enjoy the music."

"Don't worry about it, really! That's not why we're here." At North Memorial Phil, Janie and their son had blessed us with their music several times. He couldn't walk out on them there. This was dubious progress.

Phil continued to quietly play hymns and worship songs. Mom, Janie and I talked quietly and hummed along with the music. Then Phil packed up his keyboard and they left.

Mom and I found Bill in his room, lying in bed.

I gathered up my knitting bag, jackets and purses from the wide window ledge. "Let's go home."

A nurse who had just entered the room smiled understandingly. "Good plan. Go on home and get some rest." She pulled a blood pressure cuff from her pocket. "I know this is hard on you. He'll get better. This is a normal part of recovery."

"That's good to know." I sighed and turned toward my closed-eyed husband who was already making soft sleep breathing sounds. "Good night, Bill. We'll see you tomorrow. Love ya." I leaned over and gave him a quick smooch.

"Good night," he murmured.

On the way home, a billboard caught my eye. "Mom. Did you see that sign? It said that some trains of thought never reach the station." We laughed.

"Lord, please help Bill's train of thought go where it's supposed to."

I steered off one interstate and merged onto another. "His improved ring toss score was a hopeful sign." I exhaled, releasing pent-up tension. "He had the highest score. Back at North Memorial, he wouldn't even play. So this is a good sign." Bill *was* making progress. I needed to be patient.

"How do you think Jody's doing? I'm concerned about her," said Mom.

"I think she's hanging in there." Maybe I was so absorbed in my own heartache that I wasn't paying enough attention to my daughter.

"Her life is all work and seeing her dad," Mom continued. "She's young and beautiful. I'd hate to see her missing out on social life and opportunities to meet a young man."

"She has a group of friends at church. They enjoy doing things together." I remembered the circle of college-age girls and guys who talk after Sunday's service.

"That's good. Do you think there's anyone special in her life?" Mom asked.

"I've wondered the same thing but haven't wanted to pry. She's looking for someone with a heart for missions." I remembered her relationship a few years earlier with a young man who considered going into medical missions. He was likable, but something was missing from the relationship. It looked right but her heart wasn't in it.

"That's wonderful but I hope she's not narrowing her choices too much," said Mom.

"I asked her the other day if she knew anyone with the character qualities she's looking for. I promised I wouldn't pry her to tell me who if she didn't want to."

"What did she say?"

"She nodded."

"But she didn't tell you who it is?"

"Nope."

"Weren't you just dying to find out?"

"Yes, but I held my tongue."

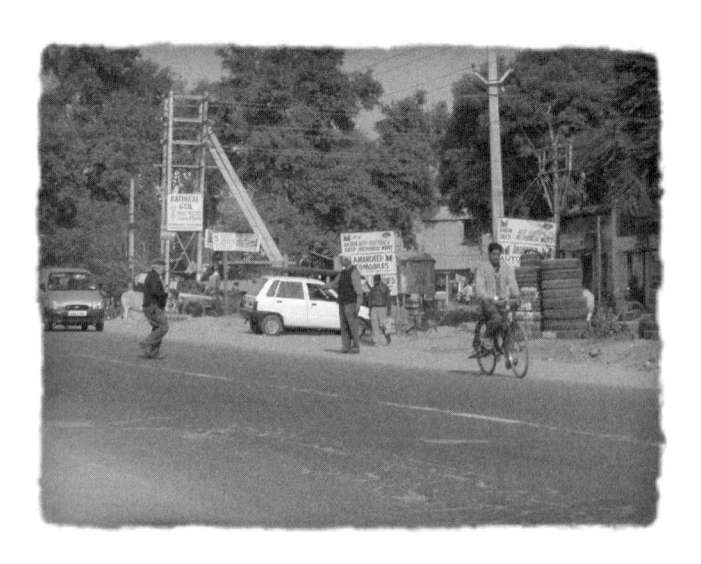

Manna in the Wilderness

THE NEXT MORNING, I awakened to sun streaming in the window. The gloom of several consecutive cloudy days had lifted. After a quick trip to the bathroom, I pulled out my Bible and devotional book which directed me to Luke 22:39-46. Jesus was facing something far worse. He was to be crucified soon. Instead of running away, he released himself into his Father's hands, saying, "Yet not my will, but yours be done." As he did so, an angel came to strengthen him.

Would Bill ever be the same again? During previous hospitalizations, he appreciated my companionship. Now I wondered if it was worth the effort and time just to chase him around the big round room. I couldn't imagine a full evening at home. *What did I do before life became abnormal?*

I relished emails but there were exceptions such as, "I've been thinking and praying about Bill's situation. He might recover faster if he were at home and in familiar surroundings." Yes, but… They hadn't seen him. *Am I a horrible spouse for not wanting him home now?*

How would I manage him, making sure he didn't escape?

What if he found the keys and attempted to drive?

What if he were incontinent and wet the bed?

What *was* ahead for us? Would he relate as a husband again or would he remain an overgrown toddler? I doubted that he would let me mother him. Yet, I needed to accept the possibility.

God, help us!

Bump on the Road

Jesus urged the disciples to pray, even though they were weary from sorrow. He had told them to pray so that they wouldn't be tempted. What were their temptations? Were they tempted to give up and act as though they never knew Jesus? Most likely their feelings were like mine–fear, anger, discouragement, hopelessness, self-pity.

Before the accident I fretted over trivia. Now as Bill groped in confusion, I was changing. This was too big for me to handle alone. I needed God's help more than ever. Weeds of striving, imagined rejection, preconceived ideas, selfish desires, and dependence on others were being yanked out by the root. Life would not be the same again, regardless of how much Bill recovered.

After Bill had completed seminary, we lived in Northern Minnesota where the forest was so dense that it was easy to get lost. Difficulties and dangers lurked. Later we lived in dry, wide-open Montana where trees and rivers were sparse. God promised to provide a way in the wilderness, providing refreshment. Bill's mind was a wilderness with inklings of life here and there.

Now we were in a wilderness through which God had promised to make a way. God, the creator of everything, calls forth rivers and life in any wilderness so that men will see and know that He is God, even in Bill's injured brain.

I returned my Bible and journal to the bedside table and slid off the bed. Time to get going.

In the kichen, I picked up a three panel card which had arrived in the mail. The inside was a watercolor painting of potted plants, waiting to go in a garden. A couple of empty broken pots lay on their sides, their contents had been transplanted. Would new life come from Bill's brokenness? Springtime is a time of hope and new growth that follows the hardships of winter. Would we survive, grow and bear fruit?

God was big enough to find a place for Bill until he could return to us. I felt my roots reaching deeper into God's soil to find water there.

That night, Jody returned home from work as Mom and I snacked on toast. Remembering Bill's improved appearance, I thanked Jody for trimming his hair that day.

"It was hilarious." She dropped her purse on the table and shrugged off her coat. "He had asked me to bring the clippers and haircutting scissors so I did." She filled a large glass with water and sat down. "I showed him the clippers and stuff. Then he sat down, pulled up his shirt and held out the feeding tube from his tummy. He thanked me for bringing the scissors and asked me to cut off the tube."

"Oh no!" I looked at Mom and we both laughed. "So what did you do?"

"I said that I couldn't do that but told him that I wanted to cut his hair. He agreed to it. I think he still thought I was going to cut the tube. Anyway, he let me put the cape on him and give him a haircut."

"You did a great job. He looks so much better."

"Thanks. I sped through it in case he got antsy before I finished. When I told him we were all done and took away the cape, he pulled up his shirt again. I told him I couldn't because I had to go to work. He nodded and didn't say anything else."

"Good for you."

"Oh yeah, remember how Dad ignored Bob and Karan when they visited last night?" said Jody.

"Yes, he acted like he didn't even know them," I replied.

"Today, when I was there, he asked me where Bob and Karan were. It was so cool!"

"That's interesting. I guess he's more aware than he lets on," I replied.

Bump on the Road

Jody went to the living room and returned with a book. It was a compilation of my dad's sermons published by his church after his death. "I've been reading your dad's sermons. This spoke to me. Can I read something to you?"

She opened to a bookmark and began reading. "The most meaningful moments of my life have not been moments of Utopian bliss. So I wonder about a system of values and a concept of destiny that assumes that absence of suffering, absence of adversity and absence of struggle are the ultimate good."

Turning some pages, she continued. "Suffering is the price of freedom, the price of a moral universe, the price of the power of decision, the price of character and the price of our deepest, highest joy."

"Wow," said Mom. "That's powerful."

"I've been enjoying your dad's sermons. It helps me feel like I know my other grandpa a little at least." She sighed. "I've missed out on knowing your parents because they died before I was born. I hope my kids can know my dad for who he really is."

She glanced around. "Whose white car is that out there?"

"I think it's going to be mine," I said.

Mom chimed in. "Your mom heard that it was for sale so she pursued it." She patted me on the arm. "Your mom is even wheeling and dealing cars now."

I laughed. "We have four derelict cars that need a dad to keep them going." I took another bite of toast. "I would like to get rid of these and get each of us one that's dependable."

"That's for sure," said Jody. "I worry about breaking down on the side of the road without Dad being able to come help."

"Joel thought it was a good idea, too," I said. "He offered to help find buyers. Otherwise, he would be stuck keeping our cars going for us."

"Cool." Jody's smile turned into a frown. "What about Dad? The brown Olds was kind of Dad's pride and joy. Will he wonder what happened to his car?"

"That's true. He'll probably ask about it one of these days." Though the Olds had gone over 200,000 miles, its velvety interior still gave a comfy ride. "Maybe we need to loan it to someone rather than getting rid of it. It feels strange and almost wrong to buy a car by myself. We've always done it together."

Though eight years old, the white Honda seemed new. It felt right as I drove it that day.

By the end of the week, the Honda was mine.

Friday, April 23, I emailed a progress report.

> For the first time in a while, I can say that Bill seems better. The therapist said that he was compliant today and had made a 180 degree turn. Looking at our photo album with Jody this noon, he saw a picture of Deanna (our granddaughter) and read the label identifying her. He said he missed her. Tonight, we took her to visit. He smiled broadly, a first since the accident, and said she had grown. He played Koosh ball with us and even laughed. He asked about the remodeling project at church. We filled him in. Then, he asked if anything was happening with plans for a Saturday night service! This was in the idea stage right before his accident. Now Saturday night services have begun. Remembering and mentioning specific areas in the building, he asked where it was held. He then asked how I was doing and if I was working. When we left, he waved goodbye. It was so encouraging to see Bill's fog lift.

At last, Bill's thoughts expanded beyond the confines of Bethesda. Our church had recently completed an around-the-clock prayer vigil for Bill's restoration. God hadn't forgotten us.

Bump on the Road

I remembered a promise that I had read during a dark moment. God had said "Do not fear, for I am with you; do not be dismayed, for I am your God. I will strengthen you and help you; I will uphold you with my righteous right hand." (Isaiah 41:10)

God isn't going to let us down.

ಌ

Mom, Bill and I were seated at a table when Bill looked up and waved. "There's Gordy and Jana," he said. Pastor Gordy and his wife Jana had entered the unit and were walking toward us.

Jana smiled and patted him on the shoulder. "Hi Bill. You're looking good."

Gordy shook Bill's hand and scooted two more chairs up to the table. "How are you, Bill?"

"Okay," Cocking his head toward his room, Bill continued. "I'm tired of being in there. I've been there all day."

Gordy chuckled. "I would be tired of it, too!"

"How are things going at church?" Bill asked.

They stayed about 15 minutes. Bill's attention faded in and out and, at times, he nodded off to sleep. Though we weren't talking about anything very complicated, I knew he was having difficulty keeping up.

"Bill, you're looking tired." Gordy stood and Jana followed suit. "We should leave so you can rest."

Jana squeezed Bill's hand. "You're doing so well. Much better than the last time we saw you a couple of weeks ago."

"I agree," said Gordy. "Keep up the good work!"

After they left, I asked a nurse for a progress report.

"He's doing okay but sleeps only about 50-80% of the night. The rest of the time, he wanders into other patients' rooms."

"Oh no." *Why was there always something negative when it seemed that Bill was getting better?*

"The doctor prescribed medication to help him sleep. So we're starting that today." She looked again at the chart in her hand. "We've increased the dosage of the medication that helps with alertness. Also, we started giving his meds by mouth today."

"That's good. How did he do?"

"He took them fine. No problem, but then he kept asking about getting something through the tube."

"Since he's eating well and taking his pills orally, can he get rid of the tube now?" Every little step toward normal life was movement toward Bill's release from imprisonment.

"We need to wait a little longer to make sure he does okay. It doesn't hurt to leave it there for now."

Bill snoozed while sitting in a *Jerry* chair, a recliner with wheels. Then I rolled him off the closed unit to the adjoining room. Three months had passed since Bill's accident. I looked out the window toward the state capitol. Lime green buds laced the trees. *Is spring coming to Bill's brain too?* I hoped that taking him outside would help. Spring. The season of new life. *Lord, let new life come for Bill, too. Please.*

A few days later, Mom and I arrived to see Bill and another patient sitting at a table with a jigsaw puzzle between them.

"Look, Mom, he's doing a ..."

"Bill! No!" I grabbed his hand as a puzzle piece disappeared into his mouth. "Don't eat that!" I rolled Bill, *Jerry* chair and all, toward Mo.

"Bill put a puzzle piece in his mouth!"

Mo expertly coaxed Bill to spit it out. I marveled at how easily and calmly Mo managed the situation.

"Here, Bill. I brought you a piece of cheesecake." I hoped this treat would distract him.

He ate it immediately but asked for the puzzle. "I need to finish. It's my responsibility."

Bump on the Road

"It's okay. Someone else is taking care of it."

He looked around, shaking his head as he studied the table where the puzzle had been. By then, someone had put it away.

Except for when he took a brief nap, he perseverated about the puzzle all evening. He would not think about anything else.

"I know this is distressing but he is making progress. It takes time but he'll be all right eventually," said Mo.

Bill's vocabulary was returning and he talked more clearly. At times he laughed, often at the frustration of no one understanding his current matter of urgency. Visits became encouraging and discouraging, humorous and sad, easier and challenging. The ebb and flow kept us in suspense.

I wondered what had happened to the glimpse of clarity the previous Friday. His questions had been so encouraging. This week, his confused mind drove him daily in one strange pursuit or another. He was frustrated with us for not helping.

"I need to have access into here." Bill stood by a locked door. "Where are the keys? There is a choir in here. I saw them earlier and I need to find them."

"There's no choir in there, Bill. It's just fuses or something." Taking Bill gently by the arm, a nurse tried to distract him.

"Can you open this door to show Bill that there isn't anything in there?" I asked.

"We can't," she replied. "Only the maintenance people have keys for it."

Holy Spirit, You live in Bill. Please infuse his mind so that he has power, love and a sound mind as promised in II Timothy 1:7!

In spite of the confusion, there were glimmers of hope and progress. He now takes medications orally, cooperated with nurses checking vitals, dressed himself, and said things such as "love you" and "good night." He kissed me often though his expression remained flat.

Another Move

A MONTH AFTER Bill's move to Bethesda, we sat at a large table for family meeting. Therapists, a neuro-psychologist, the social worker, the hospital chaplain, and a nurse were present.

Sherry, the social worker, began. "William has improved. He is progressing with tasks that he initiates or in response to stimuli."

As if to quell hopes, the speech pathologist spoke. "Unfortunately, he still isn't responding very well to verbal stimulus. This includes answering questions or following directives. For example, he doesn't brush his teeth when we tell him to, but he will if the toothbrush is given to him or set out. He'll put on clothes when we give them to him, but not when we tell him to go get dressed."

"He's talking more and asking about life outside of here."I said.

"That's good," said the neuro-psychologist. "However, his conversations are still based on what he's thinking about and not in response to what is going on. In other words, it's when it's his initiative rather than coming from another."

"Oh. I see." Though I agreed, I felt that his recent interest in life outside marked significant improvement.

"Bill's progress has slowed again," said Sherry. She looked at the others and they nodded in agreement. "We need to help you prepare for an altered life style. So that you aren't suddenly left helpless without insurance coverage, you should look into medical assistance now for long-term care."

"What are we supposed to do?" I panicked. "We can't handle him at home yet. Not like this!"

Bump on the Road

"We're not expecting you to do that," said Sherry. "A nursing home would take him and provide therapies at a slower pace. We can help you find one."

That dreaded word again. A nursing home. "Would insurance cover expenses there?"

"Yes, as long as he makes progress."

"What if he doesn't?" I was afraid to ask, fearing the answer.

"That's why you need to get the ball rolling for medical assistance. Because of the brain injury he would probably qualify."

"When would he come home, then?"

"He'd probably go to a group home." she answered.

He would come home after that. I wasn't ready to accept the idea of his not returning to a normal life.

"Isn't all this change going to be hard on him?" Mom asked. "He's already confused!"

The doctor and nurse exchanged looks. "I think we can try putting Bill in the step-down wing to help him make the transition. He'll wear a wander alert band, which would sound an alarm when he attempts to wander off."

Sherry recommended an appointment with an agency that helps families of brain injured patients. The first session would be free. She said we needed to look into *conservatorship*. Seeing my puzzlement, she said that this agency would help us understand.

Following Sherry's directive, I made an appointment for Mom and me with the firm she recommended. Though I didn't understand why, it sounded important. So much of dealing with brain injury was foreign. Staying in the dark was not an option. The hospitals would not take care of Bill and guide us forever. Eventually we would be on our own.

We drove to a southern suburb for our appointment. A receptionist led us to the office of a gray-haired gentleman, seated behind a large wooden desk. He rose and shook our hands, introducing himself. "Please have a seat and tell me what brings you here."

Another Move

"I'm not sure, but my husband is at Bethesda with a brain injury and his social worker said we should meet with you."

He chuckled and smiled. "I understand. I imagine this is very overwhelming."

At his prompting, I told the story of Bill's accident and recovery so far.

He explained that family members of brain-injured people often need to take measures to protect their finances and to secure the most help for future needs. "When a husband or wife has a severe brain injury, we help the spouse set up conservatorship. It provides legal protection to prevent the injured spouse from writing checks or making decisions that would put their finances in jeopardy."

I hadn't thought about that possibility. His checkbook and credit cards were safely stashed at home, thirty minutes from his current residence in a locked unit.

"We help families go through the legal process of removing the injured spouse's privilege to sign legal documents, authorizing one such as yourself to be the conservator."

Lord, wouldn't it be much easier to restore Bill?

He talked about applying for disability. Julie and Sherry had already explained that Bill wouldn't be eligible to receive the typical benefits because he had opted out of social security when he was a full-time pastor. Now we regretted this choice of 15 years earlier. When I explained this to the man, he could only offer sympathy.

₰

May 4, Bill was moved to the "step down" wing next to the locked unit. Though still closely monitored, he wouldn't be locked into the area. Celebrating this change, Mom and I joyfully walked

Bump on the Road

down the corridor to the nurses' station. Surely now Bill would show that he was improving and that their assessment was wrong.

When I introduced myself and our reason for being there, the woman behind the desk frowned. "Your husband has been trying to leave the unit ever since he arrived." She looked toward her left where Bill paced. "He's been hovering around the elevators trying to get on. Doors open only to let staff get off. However, he stands there and waits. When a door opens, he makes a run for it. Fortunately, he hasn't made it in time. Not yet, anyway."

"Maybe we can talk him into staying in his room." Where had that confidence come from?

She nodded though she appeared to doubt my wishful thinking.

Mom and I escorted Bill to his room. This room was smaller and looked like a regular hospital room.

"Bill, this is a pleasant room. Let's set your things out and make it look homey." I reached down to start unpacking one of the bags sitting on the floor.

He appeared to be uneasy. "I need to change the sheets on the bed."

"The sheets are fine. Besides, the staff takes care of that." I reached for his hand as he started out the door.

We trailed behind as he walked the U-shaped corridors, ending up by the elevators again.

"Let's sit here." I motioned to three nearby chairs. "Here are some magazines, Bill. Let's look at these. Okay?"

Bill brushed the magazines aside and studied the elevator buttons. "One. Two. Three. Five. Six. Seven. It doesn't have four! What's wrong with it?" He sighed in exasperation. "I need to go to fourth floor to change my sheets."

"Your sheets are fine. Besides, we're on fourth floor." I grew increasingly frustrated.

He shook his head. "I need to go back to my room on fourth floor and change the sheets."

"We're still on fourth floor. Just a different part. You're getting better so you don't need to be in the same place."

He stood.

I took his hand. "Just relax."

He exhaled heavily and sat momentarily before rising again.

Mom and I followed him on another loop through the halls. He stopped by a shelf of linens. "Are these sheets?" he asked.

I blocked his arm but he pushed my hand aside. I relented, realizing that he might be satisfied if he felt he could do something to help.

Though I had expected Bill to be confused by the change, I hadn't imagined he would *want* to go back to the locked area!

Eventually we maneuvered him back to his room. He figured out which switch worked what lights and initiated a three-way hug with Mom and me. Assuming he was beginning to adjust, we said goodbye and left.

The next morning, Sherry called. "The good news is that the feeding tube was removed this morning. The procedure was done in his room. He consented and cooperated nicely. However, he's back in the locked unit."

"Why?"

"He attempted getting on the elevators all evening. At one point, he resisted an employee. Finally, at midnight, they returned him to the locked unit. Once in familiar surroundings again, he finally went to sleep."

"Oh." Why did Bill have to make it so hard on himself?

"Bill seems to have difficulty with change. We probably won't attempt it again. Otherwise, it would be too confusing for him, moving him within Bethesda and again soon to another place."

"So what does this mean?"

"Unless he improves significantly in the next day or two, he will need to go to a locked unit at a nursing home. Probably within a week."

Bump on the Road

"Does this mean he'll be with all old people with ..."

"Yes, he'll probably be with aging people who have dementia until he gets less confused."

Oh God. Help! Won't he get more confused in the company of declining brains?

☙

With a heavy heart, I rang the bell for admittance into the locked unit that evening. Why was Bill so stubborn?

The tiny nurse, who had reassured me the first day, let us in. Seeing this familiar face helped take the edge off the disappointment of Bill's retreat to the locked ward.

"I'm sorry it didn't work for your husband in the other area," she said. "He slept well after he came here last night and has been doing fine ever since."

She continued talking as we walked. "Bill cooperated with having his feeding tube removed today. He's eating well and should do fine without it. He's in his room."

Bill smiled when he saw us. "Hi. They finally let me come back to my room last night." He shook his head and laughed dryly. "Crazy."

I didn't know what to say. I had hoped this move would be the sign of progress that insurance needed. Nonetheless, he seemed more content than the night before.

He sat down. "Is it time to go have the procedure?"

"What procedure?" I asked.

"Taking out the tube." He pointed at the large bandage taped to his belly.

"It's all done." I sat by him on the bed. "You don't have the tube anymore." I smiled as broadly as I could. "They took it out this morning."

Another Move

"When are they going to come and get me? I need a shower before my procedure. Father," he prayed, "please help me during this procedure."

He persisted until a nurse squeezed him into the shower schedule though it wasn't his normal shower day. Mom and I went downstairs to visit the vending machines.

Clean from his shower, Bill continued asking when they were going to take him downstairs. Mom picked up a songbook the chaplain had left for Bill and started singing familiar hymns. I joined in and so did Bill. He settled down briefly.

ಸಾ

Jody stopped at my office the next day. "I have a little time before going to work so I came by to tell you about Dad. He was doing really well! We talked about many things. He even asked what had happened and why he was there!"

"Really. We've been trying to tell him."

"I know." She shrugged off her jacket. "It was like a light turned on. So I told him the whole thing."

"That's great!" I had been longing for him to ask. "Did he seem to understand?"

"I think he got part of it, but it's hard to tell." She pulled her hair into a pony tail and released it. "He asked me to write it down so I started. I left the paper there so you can write, too. I think you remember everything better than I do."

"I don't know about that, but I'd be glad to write it down. Anything to help him reconnect." I hoped Bill's improvement lasted until I got there.

"Another thing was that he introduced me to all the staff people, calling them by name." She plopped her purse on the floor and sat in a chair across from my desk. "He talked about therapy, complaining about the stupid games they play there."

Bump on the Road

"Hmmm. I *wondered* if he was just being stubborn. Maybe he understands more than anyone realizes."

"The nurse explained that doing the therapies would help him get better."

"Good for her. Did he respond?"

"Hard to know." She shifted in the chair. "Oh. I wanted to tell you that Ben Selin called me last night and asked if I wanted to go out for coffee tomorrow night."

I studied her expression trying to discern her feelings. "That sounds like fun. Are you happy about it?"

She smiled and nodded. "I wonder what will come of this. We've been friends for quite awhile, hanging out together at youth group and stuff. This sounds more like a date."

"That's cool. I'll be interested in hearing how it goes." Recently I had noticed that he was often in her circle of friends after church.

"Me too." She stifled a full-fledged grin.

We talked some more about her dad and then she left.

A bit later, a nurse called. "Your husband is doing well, talking continuously."

"Good." I was eager to finish work so I could go before he reverted. I hoped that this improvement wasn't going to be short-lived like his previous steps forward.

"However, he is still requesting keys for the two locked doors as if he's trying to escape the unit."

"Oh." This wasn't good. I wondered why everyone thought he was doing so well if he was still obsessing over the keys.

"Are you coming to see him today?"

"Yes, Mom and I'll be there around six."

"Good. I'm glad you're coming. Maybe you can distract him. Give him something else to think about."

Oh. This sounded like the same old challenge. Jody's report was good so maybe today would be different. "We'll try."

"Good. We'll bring a VCR into his room. If you have some family videos, bring them in. I think he might be ready to start making some connections with his past."

After a quick supper, Mom and I headed to Bethesda.

The nurse was right. Bill insisted that he must have the keys. According to him, a children's choir awaited behind the doors.

Bill's nurse wheeled a VCR and TV cart into his room and showed us how to use it. We managed to occupy him briefly with movies of ourselves and grandchildren. Though he recognized the kids, he lost interest quickly.

"How can I do my job if I don't have the keys to open these doors?" Bill stood and sighed. "I don't understand what my role is in this place and what I should be doing."

Just then, our Indian friend, Chander, arrived. "Bill. *Kidha* – How are you?"

"*Tek ha* – okay," said Bill.

"*Vadayah* – Very good." Chander chuckled. "You remember Punjabi! Getting ready to go back to India, aren't you my buddy." Chander patted Bill on the shoulder. "Are they taking good care of you here?"

"I guess so but they keep locking my bathroom door so I can't go. They also serve used meat." He shook his head and released a short dry laugh.

Then Bill talked of plans for a trip to India, searching his memory for the name of a man with whom he plannied to travel. He asked Chander if he had started using his boat yet. He mentioned mutual Indian friends and was surprised when Chander said that these friends had visited Bill a couple of times. As Chander prepared to leave, Bill requested prayer together. I was amazed by how lucid Bill could be one minute and how quickly he regressed the next. My hope bobbed up and down like a buoy on a storm-tossed lake. When he prayed or talked about God, he was most like his former self.

Getting Closer

JODY RETURNED from her coffee date with Ben Selin and settled beside me on the bed.

"How was it?" I asked.

"Interesting. We didn't really talk until we were in the parking lot."

"So, you just sat there and ate?"

"Oh, we talked but not about anything significant." She pulled off her socks and tossed them to the floor. "When we went outside to our cars, he asked what I thought of courtship."

This was getting interesting. I stuffed my pillow against the head board and sat up against it.

She continued. "I took this to mean he was interested in a special relationship with me so I asked him how he wanted to start. He turned red and hedged around. Then he said he was wondering what I thought of that concept versus dating."

"I bet you felt stupid."

"I did, but then he said that what he really wanted to ask was about being more than casual friends. He was trying to see where I was at in the relationship. When I responded like that, he realized I was interested. So... We decided to start seeing each other."

"That's great! Are you excited?"

"Yeah, but I'm reluctant to let my heart go if he doesn't have a vision for missions. I don't want him going into it because of me. You know?" She studied me to see if I understood.

Getting Closer

I nodded. "I think you need to listen to your heart. The last relationship seemed right because he had a similar vision. All that lined up. Yet, you didn't connect in other ways."

"That's for sure! It's so confusing." She shifted to her side. "I sure miss Dad's input. This is such an important time in my life. Dad has always helped me sort things out."

I squeezed her hand. "I'm sure you do."

"In two days, Ben leaves for Camp DuNord where he'll work this summer. I think it's about six hours away." She sighed. "We'll write, and he'll probably come home a few times. He did last year. I told him that I don't want to pressure him into missions. So he's going to fast and pray for the first two weeks, seeking God's vision for his life. Then, we'll see what's next."

"That sounds wise."

"We were thinking that Ben could visit Dad with me when he's here. That way they can get to know each other as much as possible."

"That's a good idea." I adjusted my pillow. "Dad was extra talkative tonight. He asked a bunch of questions like where our home was, where I went when I left at night, and how to call me."

"That's cool!"

"Then he asked about his car."

Her eyebrows went up. "Really?"

"I explained that we had lent it to Pastor Gordy's son since we didn't need it right now."

"Was he okay with that?"

"I think so." I sighed. "I'm sure glad we didn't sell it! Hopefully, this was easier for him to accept because someone is able to use it. He's always been generous with his things."

"I didn't feel peace about getting rid of it either," said Jody. "He would have felt manipulated by our selling his car."

"Then, right before I left, I told him that we were going to take him to an appointment with the surgeon at North Memorial

143

next week. He started to fidget as though we were getting ready right then. I tried to explain, but couldn't convince him. He looked puzzled and forlorn as I said goodbye. I didn't know how to console him."

∽

The next day, two friends came to Bethesda while I was there. It was getting warmer so I thought that fresh air would benefit Bill. Besides, going outside would be a good practice run for the upcoming doctor's appointment.

I retrieved Bill's winter jacket from the closet. "Bill. We're going to go outside. For a walk." I guided his arms into the sleeves. He mumbled something about the zipper. To my dismay, I discovered that the zipper pull was gone. I managed to zip it part way.

Once outside, I pointed up the street. "Bill, see the state capitol. It's right there." I think I was more impressed with its closeness than Bill was. He mumbled something that I didn't hear so I asked him to repeat.

"Where are some scissors? I need to cut these straps," said Bill. He tugged on the cloth bands fastening him to the wheelchair. "I need to go back."

"Let's go around a bit. This is your first time outside. Let's enjoy it." I faked enthusiasm. For all the talk of his trying to escape the unit, why was he unhappy about being outside? "Are you warm enough, Bill?"

"It's cold out here. I want to go back."

"Okay." I turned the chair around toward Bethesda. Though it was May 7, the air remained damp and chilly.

Back inside, Bill's occupational therapist commented that this had been a good day for Bill. He had cleaned up and dressed on his own without coaching.

Getting Closer

The following evening, Joel and Bridget brought five year old Deanna with them. I arranged with the nurse to take Bill into a small lounge next to the locked unit. Joel's fishing stories piqued his Dad's interest. Bill laughed as he envisioned Joel's dog fishing.

Bill asked if the fish mobile hanging overhead would light up. Did he remember the large lighted aquariums at North Memorial?

"This place has a different sort of culture," he commented.

Culture? It seemed that my husband's mission vocabulary was returning. I waited for further comments.

"I didn't eat supper tonight because they keep serving *used meat*," he said.

The beef noodle casserole left on his plate didn't look very exciting but I attempted to defend the institution's cuisine. "It was *ground* beef, Bill. Hamburger. They wouldn't serve *used* meat here."

Whereas a great influx of people had come to see Bill at North Memorial, the number of visitors had diminished to a few. Bill seemed to enjoy seeing people now, so I asked friends to visit. Glimmers of the real Bill were getting brighter. Finally.

John had been overseas again for a few weeks and visited Bill after his return. He noticed significant changes. Suspecting that people were tired of hearing from me only, I asked John to write the May 11 update:

> It was very encouraging to see Bill regaining memories. He talked at length about past church experiences, the joy of having home groups, remembering one by one who was part of the groups, (sometimes groping for names, but recognizing the names when reminded). He smiled, laughed, and showed his old humor many times during the evening. Sometimes, he would get on a track of thought that was rational, but seemed like a record that skipped a little. His vocabulary was rich, and he spoke of things I knew were close to his heart.

Bump on the Road

I felt strongly: "Bill is coming home…" The conversations were at his initiative, and it didn't go so well when we initiated a subject, but…so what! He's "steering his own ship back into port." (Like the doctor in India who told Cheryl how the recovery would be…a ship returning to port, but needing to visit islands along the way before final arrival.)

There is still a long way to go, many places for him to visit on the way in…but, I felt strongly tonight that he's "coming home" on the inside. By God's grace, in God's time, he'll also be home again with family, friends, church, and ministry. That's what I believe, not just because of my time with him tonight, but because of God's blood covenant with Bill. And Cheryl. And their family. And all of us. By God's grace and healing power, FULL RECOVERY is what I believe in my heart about Bill.

༄

The day came for our venture across the city. Joel, Jody, Mom and I drove through rain and thick commuter traffic, arriving at Bethesda at eight in the morning. Bill was dressed, wearing his jacket, and waiting.

"Bill, we're going to take you to see the surgeon at North Memorial. He's the one who did your surgery and he wants to see how you're doing now."

"Who?" Bill asked.

"The neurosurgeon at North Memorial," I answered.

"How are we going there?"

"We'll go in the car I bought. You get to see it today."

"What about my car?" Bill asked.

"We lent it to Pastor Gordy's son, Andrew. He needed a car to use and, since you don't need it right now, we let him use it." I shifted feet nervously. "I hope that's okay."

Bill nodded.

Thankfully Bill's generous nature was still intact.

We were nervous about how Bill would respond outside the controlled environment to which he had adjusted. We contained him in a wheelchair that Joel pushed out to the parking ramp.

All of us went – Joel, Mom, Jody and me. Jody and I hemmed Bill in the middle of the back seat, making sure the doors were locked. Wedged between us, escape wouldn't be easy. Throughout the half-hour ride, he asked where we were going, what road we were on, and what direction we were headed.

Upon arrival at North Memorial, Joel let us out at the hospital entrance. Jody and I each grabbed a hand and led Bill to a wheelchair in the lobby. Mom trailed behind. Once he understood what he was supposed to do, he sat in the chair. I pushed him to the familiar CT scan area.

I had barely finished my coffee from the kiosk when a nurse brought Bill to us. "We're all done, aren't we William?"

Bill nodded.

"How did it go?" I asked, remembering the exasperating times earlier when he hadn't cooperated, and they had to reschedule his CT scan.

"He did fine." She handed me a large envelope. "Here's his scan. You can take this with you to the doctor." She nodded toward the adjacent medical arts building.

So far so good. Joel wheeled Bill through an underground passage and up several levels to the surgeon's office where we crowded into a small examining room.

The doctor leaned toward Bill. "Can you tell me your name?"

"I'm William Oliver Barr," said Bill slowly as if to make sure the doctor understood.

"Good. Can you tell me where you are?" asked the surgeon.

Bill grinned and pointed to the doctor's chest. "I'm here to see you."

"That's right. Do you know today's date?"

Bill looked puzzled and then shook his head.

The doctor gestured toward the one-day-at-a-time calendar above Bill's head. "It's Wednesday, May 12, today." He stood. "Let's go take a look at these films."

Bill calmly remained seated in the examining room with Mom. Joel, Jody and I followed the doctor into the hall where he clipped the scans to a light board. "The shunts are working and things look good though there is significant damage. I expect Bill to improve for another six to nine months. Then, he will plateau where he will stay."

He unclipped the scans. "I won't need to see William unless some problems develop. Continue follow-up with the neurologist at Bethesda." The surgeon stood and shook hands with each of us. Then he turned toward me. "He is recovering well but don't expect him to return to work."

God, You can do more than that. I'm not going to stop believing in You.

∞

The next evening, Phil and Janie arrived but without the keyboard.

Bill smiled and waved when he saw them. "Hi Phil and Janie. It's good to see you."

Phil patted Bill on the shoulder and shook his hand. Janie gave him a quick side hug. "Good to see you, too!"

"Have you been able to get the tornado damage repaired yet?" Bill asked.

"You remember that? Good for you!" Phil smiled and glanced at his wife. "Yes, we had to wait several weeks because there was much wreckage in our area. They did the repairs and everything's good as new now."

"I repaired a fence for an Indian man last summer, too. It had been hit by a tornado." With accurate detail, Bill described the process. Then he changed the subject, "The surgery must have been cancelled."

"Oh yes, I'm sure it has." Was he ever going to stop expecting *the procedure*?

Now we had another challenge. I pulled an envelope from my purse. It held two checks that required Bill's endorsement for deposit—a tax refund and an insurance claim. I worried that he would spoil the checks by writing the wrong thing or in the wrong spot.

"Here, Bill, practice writing your name here." I turned over the envelope of the insurance check and pushed it toward him. Eventually, he obligingly took the pen and wrote *practice* and *write* on the envelope.

"No Bill. Write your *whole name* here—William Oliver Barr!" Phil and Janie helped coach Bill to understanding. Though it took a half hour, I left that night with both checks signed for deposit!

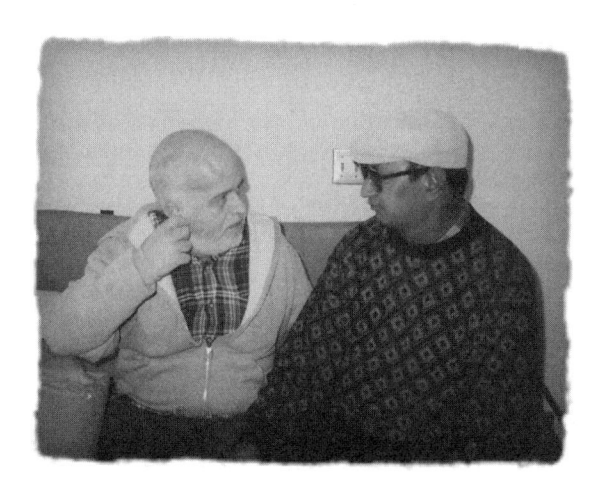

Expanding Horizons

BEN HAD BEEN GONE for a week when he called Jody. While they talked, I hung out with Mom in her room. When she got sleepy, I returned upstairs.

As I washed my face, Jody appeared in the bathroom doorway. "Ben and I had a good talk. He spent some time praying and fasting when he first got to Camp DuNord. He senses that God wants him to reach out to people and it doesn't matter where. Here or abroad. He also has a vision for leading worship. He's open to missions."

I recalled my own aversion toward missions during our first twenty-five years of marriage.

"I think that's great. God will take care of the mission thing in His way and His timing." My daughter was falling in love. I could see it in her eyes. "Even though your dad and I didn't share the same vision for years, we have been right for each other."

Though Camp DuNord was six hours away, Ben managed frequent blitz trips at least once a week. I wondered when he slept. Wanting to build a relationship with Bill, he accompanied Jody to Bethesda regularly.

"Cheryl." Bill looked at me earnestly. "I think we need to encourage Jody to fall in love with Ben. I told her about Jen's marital plans. I think Jody should get together with her to talk about how to fall in love."

"Uh huh." I didn't know what to say. I hadn't noticed any problem with Jody's ability to fall in love.

"I would like to meet with ..." He rubbed his forehead. "You know, the man who runs the camp. Where Ben is working. Maybe Jody can go there and spend some time at the camp."

I imagined contacting Brian, whom we knew but hadn't seen for several years. Would he want to take the time to visit Bill in the hospital?

Back home afterwards, I had entwined my fingers in dental floss, when Jody joined me in the upstairs landing by our bedrooms.

"I really, really miss Dad's counsel, ... you know?"

"I'm sure you do." I smiled as I remembered Bill's conversation earlier that day. "He approves of Ben. In fact, he wanted you to talk to Jen about how to fall in love."

"Oh, funny!" She laughed but grew serious again. "But I still miss his wisdom. At this point, Dad thinks that both Ben and I work at Bethesda so he thinks he's matchmaking us."

"Even in his confused state, he's supportive of this relationship." I hoped that would ease her mind. "He wants to talk to Brian about you spending time at the camp this summer."

"Really?" She giggled. "Ben and I talked about me going up for a visit. I guess I have Dad's okay to go see Ben! We thought I could go at the end of summer when I'm done with summer school."

⁓

Brother Kaushal, Indian Bible School director, emailed to say that he was planning a trip to the United States and wanted to include us in his itinerary. Though Bill was a long way from his pre-accident self, I looked forward to our Indian friend seeing Bill's improvement. I met Brother Kaushal at the airport and took him directly to Bethesda.

When Bill saw Brother Kaushal, his eyebrows went up and he pointed at the older man. "Where did you find him?"

"I picked him up at the airport. He came to visit."

Bump on the Road

Bill launched into nonstop conversation, describing experiences in India and in Minnesota with Indian friends. As long as he set the course, the conversation seemed almost normal.

"Brother, God is good. You are so much better." Brother Kaushal rotated his tan cap in his hands.

"Jody told me I was thrown from a motorcycle. In India. Tell me, what happened?"

Brother Kaushal began to describe the story in detail.

Bill retrieved a pen from his pocket. "Cheryl, write this down."

I took a yellow pad from Bill's table and took notes.

"Today I remembered something," said Bill. "It was like a dream. I was riding on a motorcycle. Then everything went black. Like I went into a hole."

"Ah, you must be remembering what you experienced as you had your accident." I was excited about this indication that his memory was returning.

Bill interrupted again and looked at me. "Why do you sleep in a different place?"

"I don't think they'll let me stay." He wasn't avoiding me anymore, but now we had a different problem.

"We can ask them to move your bed into here. There's no reason why you need to stay in a different room since you work here, too."

"I'll come visit every day."

During Brother Kaushal's visit, Ben and Jody suggested taking Bill to the zoo. It sounded doable. Brother K, Ben, Jody, and I led Bill out to my car.

I handed my keys to Ben and invited Brother Kaushal to sit in front. Bill rode in the back between Jody and me. We went about 15 minutes to Como Park Zoo. I took Bill's hand as we started walking toward the park entrance.

Bill stopped in front of a sign. "Humph. No pets allowed." He shook his head. "Pathetic. A zoo without animals."

Then he paused at another sign. "Don't feed the animals" He snorted. "What kind of zoo is this if you can't give food to the animals? Don't they need food?"

Though he didn't do anything bizarre, I wondered if passers by noticed anything different about him. Several times he needed to use a restroom. I was grateful for two men to supervise him.

"We should probably go back now," said Bill.

"Are you getting tired, Dad?" asked Jody.

"I think I need to go back."

"That's fine." I took Bill's hand and steered him toward the parking lot. I was relieved that he took initiative to return to Bethesda and that our outing was incident-free.

During Brother K's visit, Pastor Gordy hosted another Indian pastor friend, Paul. After the Sunday morning service, Pastor Gordy and Paul met Brother K and me at the hospital to pray for Bill. When Bill saw Paul, his face brightened in recognition. Paul embraced Bill and said, "We have come to pray for you, Brother Bill."

"Good," replied Bill. He continued to tell about a couple from church who had visited him earlier that day, describing a miraculous answer to prayer they had experienced.

We followed a nurse to the adjoining conference room where Phil had played keyboard a few days earlier. Before we had finished settling into the chairs, Bill began to pray. "Thank You, Lord, for these Indian brothers. Please bless their ministries and work in India. Bless Pastor Gordy, his work and his family."

After he finished we looked at each other and smiled. "We came to pray for you, Bill," said Pastor Gordy, "but you prayed for us. Thank you. Can we pray for you now?"

"Yes, please do."

Bump on the Road

After all three pastors had prayed, Pastor Gordy put his hand on Bill's shoulder. "We are having a special meeting tonight at the church to pray for you some more. Brother Kaushal will speak."

That evening the sanctuary filled with friends, some of whom no longer attended our church. Jody spotted the couple which Bill had mentioned visiting him earlier that day. She described what he had said about praying for the miracle in their family.

"That's awesome," said the wife. "When we were there, we wondered if he even recognized us. He didn't say much, but we chatted with him, anyway."

Thursday evening, the day before Brother Kaushal's departure, we took photos of India trips to the hospital. Bill remembered events, places and people. His comments were clear and coherent as though nothing had happened to his brain.

After observing this interaction, two nurses said that, during Brother Kaushal's stay, they had noticed significant progress in Bill. Reflecting to a week earlier, I agreed.

"I was planning a trip to India with…" Bill looked at me and rubbed his temple. "Who was it?"

I shrugged. "I don't know."

"He was from Washington. Where's that place out west … up there where all the Punjabis live?"

"Vancouver?" I asked.

He shook his head. "Steve …. What's his last name?"

"Steve from Vancouver? I don't remember him."

He sighed and grew quiet.

With Bill's improvement new challenges surfaced. It was hard enough to convince Bill that I didn't live at Bethesda, let alone explain that he couldn't go to India sometime soon. Pre-accident Bill had been so independent and capable. I wondered if he had any idea how different he was now. Would he ever recover enough to travel abroad? I sighed. One day at a time. God gives grace when we need it. I told myself not to worry.

Bill's imminent move to another facility loomed. As my husband talked nonstop to Brother Kaushal in one room, I met with Sherry, the social worker. She had found possibilities for Bill's transfer. This was both encouraging and disheartening. The only secured units in skilled care facilities were for aging folks with dementia. Would he copy them instead of learning appropriate behavior? Why couldn't they see his progress and let him stay at Bethesda a little longer?

Then it was time to take Brother Kaushal to the airport. Bill insisted that one of us was supposed to draw blood for a test. This pre-empted a proper goodbye to our Indian friend. I was frustrated, but Brother Kaushal didn't seem concerned.

Tuesday, May 18, I was exhausted so I asked Jody to write the update.

> My dad had a good day. When I saw him this morning he spent the whole time talking, which is his favorite thing to do now. It's so exciting to listen to him and hear how he perceives things. It is very evident to me that he must have spent quite a bit of time with his Heavenly Father when he was unable to communicate with us. He is constantly talking about God's fire touching people and how everyone has some kind of ministry. He spent a long time talking about my niece, Deanna, and her ministry of playing the organ for young children. He also prays for the therapists and the nurses to be filled with the Holy Spirit's fire. God is definitely working through him even in this state of mind. I can't wait to see how God will work through him as he comes out of this.
>
> Thank you all for standing with my family during this time. I know that it has changed me dramatically along with everyone else in my family. It is so neat to see how

> God works through the difficulties in our lives to mold us into the people that He wants us to be. I consider it an honor to be going through this, because God is doing surgery on all our lives that will change us forever. Don't be afraid of hard times. Instead, look for the lessons that God has hidden inside His magnificent puzzle.

Jody's maturity was far beyond her nineteen years. What a wonderful daughter, a great ally in the valley of the shadow of death.

As I prayed and pondered, I found a promise in Isaiah 40:10-11. God has power. Yet, He loves us with tender, gentle love. *God, please carry Bill, Your lamb, close to Your heart to assure and love him.*

My devotional book took me to Psalm 25 which reminded me that, when we trust God, He doesn't put us to shame. In his weakened condition, Bill still trusts the Lord. Surely, God wouldn't leave him in a shameful way. He promises to direct the humble.

Lord, please guide us.

Monday, May 24, we completed arrangements for Bill's move to Trevilla of Golden Valley. Though he would start out on the secured floor for Alzheimer's, Bill could graduate to the short-term rehab section. Because of their focus on rehab, this was a satisfactory option.

Suspecting that Bill struggled with hearing, I asked Sherry to write a note for him, explaining his move. She did, stating that he would have treatments there and that his goal was to regain independence so he could return home. She concluded with "Congratulations!" and had attached a sheet about Trevilla with a picture of the building.

Bill read the note and smiled. "I'm going to have more therapy so I can go home eventually."

Later that day, Bill and I sat across from each other at a small table in the common area. His expression was sad and serious. "I need to ask your forgiveness. I confused you with someone on the staff here. Today I realized that she was different. I asked her to forgive me. Now I ask you to please forgive me."

Taking his hands in mine, I replied "Yes, I forgive you! I'm really glad you realized that. Thank you."

Pointing to the scar on his forehead, he asked "Is this from the accident?"

"Yes, it is. They removed part of your skull to relieve pressure on your brain. It's a scar from that."

"It's okay for you to go home and stay with Mom and Jody and for me to stay here."

"Thank you. We'll come back tomorrow and go with you to the new place."

"Let's pray together about this move," said Bill. He reached for my hand and prayed briefly.

I was relieved and glad that he understood the upcoming move so well. This was even better than I had dared to hope.

It seemed that his thinking and understanding had cleared significantly within the last 24 hours. For two months, we had been telling him that both of our sons were expecting babies. Finally, he understood and joined us in anticipation of these new grandchildren.

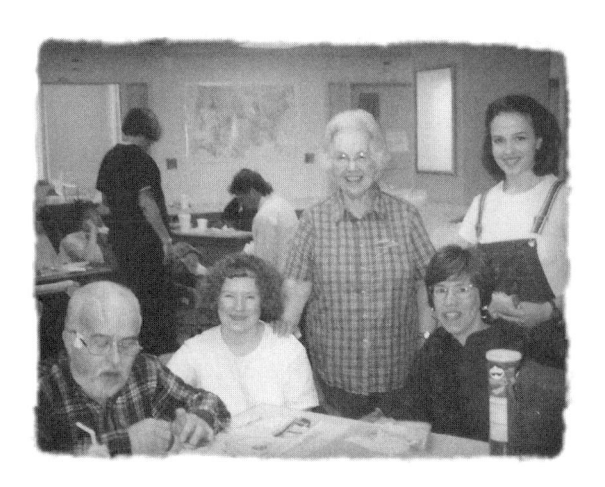

Ready to Work

JODY, JOY, MOM and I watched Bill eat his last Bethesda meal. Nurses came and went, saying goodbye. One said, "Bill has got to be the nicest man we've had. Brain injuries usually cause personality changes, making mellow people aggressive. Has he always been kind and gentle?"

"Yes, he has," I replied.

"You're fortunate," she said.

Lord, thank You for protecting Bill's personality.

We loaded up Bill and his belongings in my car and Joy's. From the shadow of the state capitol in downtown St. Paul, we drove west to Golden Valley, a western suburb of Minneapolis. Bill's head turned constantly as he attempted to read the highway signs. Repeatedly, he asked which road we were on. I almost heard the gears of his brain connecting the dots of once familiar pathways around our metro.

"Where did you say we're going?" asked Bill.

"We're going to Golden Valley," I answered. "To Trevilla. It's a skilled-care facility."

"Tre…veh…?"

"Trevilla." I wondered how many times we would need to repeat the name until Bill got it.

A half hour later, we pulled up in front of a four-story, brick building with an awning-covered sidewalk leading into the main entrance. Joy and Jody, who had followed in Joy's car, pulled up behind us. Bill and Mom got out and waited, surrounded by suitcases and bags. I parked in the "visitor" parking area. No more parking ramp fees. Yahoo!

We walked through a large lounge. Silver-haired and wrinkled people sat in paisley print vinyl wing-back chairs. A myriad of fish drifted back and forth in a large aquarium. I led the way to the receptionist desk and explained why we were there.

"I'll page the floor nurse," said the woman on the other side of the tall counter. "She'll be right with you."

Soon a woman appeared and led us to the elevator which we rode to the second floor.

Bill's new room had two beds separated by a curtain. A woman sat in a chair next to an elderly man lying in the bed closest to the window. She said that a stroke had left the man blind and unable to walk.

An African woman, Lydia, introduced herself as the charge nurse. She explained procedures, gave me forms to fill out, and took us on a tour. A bathroom with a sink and toilet was between Bill's room and the next.

"When do I have therapy?" Bill asked.

"Since you're getting settled, we'll wait to start therapy tomorrow," Lydia answered.

At last Bill was serious about therapy.

ഔ

A week after this transition, it was my birthday. We picked up Bill and went as a family to an Indian restaurant nearby. How different this was from Valentine's Day in India, three and a half months earlier! Whereas he hardly spoke then, he was now talking nonstop and animated about my birthday.

Our friend, Pal Cheema, owned the restaurant and beamed when we arrived. He waved his hand toward the far end. "Bill, do you remember building and painting these walls?"

Bump on the Road

Bill nodded and grinned. "We put up the curtains, too."

"That's right." The two men lapsed into speaking Punjabi. "You still speak Punjabi," said Pal. "That's good."

"I'm glad I still remember how."

"Yes." Pal grinned. Then he resumed his duties as we feasted. Then the family surrounded me with gifts.

Through misty eyes, I read a poem that Jody had written and framed.

There is a diamond
Who is being refined.
The Father is polishing her
Causing her to shine.

The road has not been easy
With many ruts and cracks
But the Father has carried her
Close within His heart.

This diamond is shining brighter
As the pride and selfishness fall.
She opens up her being
Surrendering it all to Him.

Though the journey is wearisome,
It is causing her to trust
In the arms of her Heavenly Father
Who is able to see the end.

This journey has become a testimony
To all who listen to her story.
As they stand with her in prayer,
The Father works in them.

Perhaps she'll never be famous,
But this diamond will never be forgotten
Amongst the hearts of her loved ones
As we listen to her story.

"I wrote it last night," said Jody.

"That blesses me so much. Thank you!" With the corner of a napkin, I wiped away tears and handed the poem to Bill.

"I felt like God gave me that," said Jody. "I hope you don't mind but I emailed it to the update list and told them it was your birthday."

"I *wondered* how so many knew about my birthday! I've gotten lots of cards."

My wonderful daughter thinks of everything.

My husband adapted to his new surroundings more easily than I expected he could. Engaging in pastoral mode, he endeavored to care for others and asked God to restore his own mind so that he could minister again. Describing what he did in therapy, he said that it would help his brain work better. One day he helped make sweet rolls. They discussed safety issues and "what would you do if..." and worked on visual memory by having him copy drawings of shapes. I thanked God silently that Bill finally understood the purpose of all this.

Bit by bit, Bill put together pre-accident memories and events. "How was your visit in Holland after you left India?" he asked one day.

Clear thinking alternated with confusion. For several days, he thought his bathroom was unavailable and that he needed to find another. Once he took us downstairs to the therapy area because he knew of a bathroom there.

When his conversation muddled, I attempted redirecting to a different subject. That was almost impossible. It was as though his train of thought had only one destination.

For the first time in a family meeting, therapists reported acceptable improvement. Progress at last! Using the ship approaching harbor analogy, Bill had reached another island the

Bump on the Road

day before his move to Trevilla. Prayers for the transition were answered, even beyond our hopes.

"We're working on *path finding*," said the speech therapist. "This means orienting him to where things are so that he can figure out where he is so that he doesn't get lost. Until he masters this, he needs to stay on the locked unit."

Soon after this positive meeting, I noticed that Bill coasted into a rest stop. He seemed discouraged, struggling to understand what was being said and what was taking place around him. His perception told him one thing when reality was quite different. I purposed to take him outdoors regularly, whether to walk to the nearby Dairy Queen, sit in the park area, or walk around the building. I hoped this would help clear his mind and quicken his interests.

To expand his horizons, I took him to a nearby McDonald's. Dipping French fries in ketchup and eating a burger, Bill said, "It's nice to do these normal things. There was even a drier for hands in the bathroom."

Ah, almost like old times.

An Indian woman walked in, saw us, and came to our table. "You're Bill Barr, aren't you?"

"Yes, I am." Bill studied her.

"Remember me?" She waited.

He nodded hesitatingly.

"I'm Shashi. You were going to come to our house."

I piped up. "I remember that and wondered how I could contact you and tell you what happened. He was in a motorcycle accident in India."

"Oh no!" She frowned. "When?"

"Almost five months ago. January 26," I said.

"So so terrible. I'm so sorry."

"He's been in the hospital and now he's at Trevilla nearby."

She glanced at her watch. "I need to go to work but it was so good to see you. Come to my house sometime. Okay?"

"Yes, we will."

Bill looked at his left hand and then at his right. "Where's my wedding ring?"

"In India your whole body was so swollen that they couldn't remove the ring so they had to cut it off. I want to take you to a store to get another one."

"Okay."

Two days later, he asked about it again. Having put the damaged ring in my purse, I took it out to show him. "I found a store nearby where we can buy one exactly like the one you had."

The next day, Mom and I took Bill to the jeweler and ordered a new ring that looked like his old one. Every day after that, Bill asked about his ring. Finally, a week later, it arrived. He seemed pleased and relieved.

Bit by bit, we reintroduced Bill to his life.

Noticing occasional pet visitors, I loaded our Schnauzer into his crate for a ride to Trevilla.

When Bill saw the dog, he asked, "What's he doing here?"

"We brought him to visit you. Remember him?"

"Oh." Bill nodded slightly.

We went for a short walk around the facility with our dog stopping frequently to sniff. After Bill's apathetic response to his canine visitor, we didn't bother again.

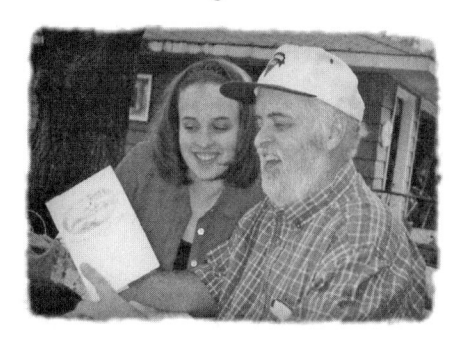

Another Plateau

MID-JUNE, the Trevilla social worker called. According to the therapy department, Bill's progress had leveled off. She said that if he didn't start improving again, insurance coverage for Trevilla would discontinue on July 1.

Not again! My poor hubby. What were we to do? I listened begrudgingly as she urged me to apply for medical assistance. They would evaluate Bill's condition and, if he was certified "disabled," we would qualify for assistance in caring for him at home.

Wanting to address anything that could slow Bill's progress, I requested hearing and vision tests. Maybe there was a simple solution that would push him forward again.

In my melancholy, I identified with Psalmist David. Consumed by sorrows, David had cried out to God. In Psalm 13, David's mood shifted from despair to hope. "But I trust in your unfailing love; my heart rejoices in your salvation. I will sing to the Lord, for he has been good to me."

I appreciated David's honest relationship with his creator. He wasn't afraid to tell God his feelings. Yet, he recalled what God had done previously and acknowledged God's character of love, faithfulness and greatness.

I decided to try David's approach by focusing on how God had helped us during other crises. Bill really had come a long way, and I needed to acknowledge that.

At times, he seemed almost normal; but within seconds, he drifted again. I sought ways to anchor Bill in reality.

Another Plateau

Sitting by him on his bed I looked at him and said, "I got new glasses today. How do they look?"

Leaning toward me, he nodded. "They look good. Are they working out better and free of the problems you were having with your other ones?"

"Yes, they're good." This small glimmer of the former Bill was heartening.

"I'm supposed to take my roommate outside, but they blocked me." Bill shook his head in disgust. "This stupid thing on my ankle started screaming obscenities."

I wondered how I could ever convince him that it wasn't his responsibility to entertain his ninety-three year old roommate who seemed content to lie in bed.

Two days after my request for a hearing test, a tall man wearing dark-rimmed glasses arrived in Bill's room.

"Hello, Mr. Barr. I am Richard from audiology." He set a large black case on Bill's bedside table. "I came to do a hearing test." He shook Bill's hand. Then Bill slid his feet over the edge of the bed and stood slowly.

"We'll do it here, Mr. Barr. Just sit down on your bed."

Bill looked dubious.

Richard patted the bed. "Have a seat."

"Right here?" Bill paused and then sat slowly.

Opening his case, Richard pulled out headphones, which he placed on Bill's head. He plugged their cord into a box-shaped device with a dial on it.

"Okay, we're going to test your left ear first, then your right. Say *yes* when you hear a sound." He slowly turned the dial. I faintly heard the tone as it gradually went from low to high.

After testing both ears, Richard put away the equipment. "Mr. Barr, your ears themselves are not damaged. The only hearing loss is what's normal for someone your age."

"That's good!" Relief crossed Bill's face, then puzzlement. "I haven't been able to hear very well with this ear, though." He pointed to his left side.

"That's because your auditory perception was affected by the injury. Your brain is having difficulty processing what it hears."

Bill nodded.

Richard pointed to Bill's right ear. "Use this ear, your good ear when you talk on the phone." He paused briefly. "You'll need to develop the skill of lip reading, too."

"Would a hearing aid help?" Bill asked.

"No, because your ears themselves are fine. It's processing information that's the problem."

Turning toward me, Richard continued. "You'll need to speak clearly and slowly when communicating with Bill. Stating things three different ways helps, too. To communicate important information, write it down."

Bill described his accident and his recoupment.

The audiologist zipped his case shut and turned toward me. "The rambling monologue is a common coping mechanism for the frustration of not understanding."

I followed the audiologist into the hallway. "Thanks for your help." Not only had he verified my suspicions of audio perception challenges, he instructed Bill on how to compensate.

A week later, Bill and I went downstairs to the beauty shop. Hair care products lined part of one wall. With eyebrows twisted in puzzlement, Bill looked around. "I thought I was going to an eye doctor."

A man arose from a stool. "That's right. I come once a week to do eye exams and share the space with the beautician." He motioned toward the barber chair. "Have a seat."

Hesitatingly, Bill sat.

"I'm going to turn off the lights for a minute and take a look at your eyes."

Another Plateau

After shining a light into Bill's eyes, the optician tested Bill's vision using charts with various lenses.

"Slip your reading glasses on for me, okay? Read this with them on," said the doctor.

Bill read the chart slowly but accurately.

"Those seem to do fine. I don't think your vision has changed." He patted Bill's knee. "Way to go."

Though the results of the auditory and vision tests were favorable, they ruled out the hope of physical factors working against my husband's recovery. Hearing aids and stronger eyeglasses weren't the solution.

I begged Michelle, the social worker, to find a place for Bill on fourth floor with younger people in recovery from similar injuries. *Can't they see that his confusion is compounded by his floor mates who are more disoriented than he is?* She said they would watch for an opening on fourth floor, but wasn't very hopeful.

She encouraged us to take Bill home for occasional visits, suggesting a few hours at first and then an overnight. On Fathers' Day, I took Bill to our house for a picnic. Joel, Bridget and Deanna, Mom, Jody, Peter and Joy were all there. We grilled burgers and had several salads.

After the meal, he wanted to take a nap. At the family's urging, I laid down next to him on our bed. "Ah, this is good," he said. Immediately he dozed off. I lay beside him, thinking how natural yet odd this was.

A half hour later, he awakened. He got up, opened the closet and studied the clothes. "This is strange." He shook his head and closed the door. "I think I need to get back to Tre...valla."

Though comforted by the familiarity of home, confusion continued as an unwelcome resident wherever he was.

I was grateful for how far he had come, but the bumpy ride continued. Mutual give-and-take, emotional support, heart-to-heart conversations, and sorting out decisions had been the substance of our relationship. We were still a long way from that. Would we ever have it again? I was desperate for an infusion of the Holy Spirit's strength to take me beyond my own abilities, emotions and wisdom.

෨

June 28, we had another family meeting with the staff.

"Though we saw great progress during Bill's first week at Trevilla, he has slowed down now."

"Why do you think that is?" I asked.

"I'm not sure," answered the speech therapist. "You may not see much progress beyond this now."

"He seems to struggle in his present environment with all the mixed up people around him. I think he gets confused by things he hears them saying, don't you?" I was grasping for possible solutions, wanting him to surprise everyone again as he had before.

"Yes, he'll probably be better in some ways at home but other confusing issues will come up." The therapist rolled her pencil slowly between her fingers. "He'll improve a bit at first but, ultimately, there won't be much change after going home."

The case manager said, "We talk with insurance companies regularly about the progress of our patients and do all we can to keep our people on insurance." She handed me copies of Bill's medical reports. "You should apply for medical assistance right away so that he can get on immediately when insurance stops covering therapies. You need copies of last year's taxes, recent bank statements, and documentation of expenses."

I hated searching for things but, at least, I was beginning to remember where to look for important papers. I wondered if I would eventually crack from these stressors.

Somehow I found what I needed.

Another Plateau

The next day I carried an inch-high stack of papers into the Anoka County Government Center to meet with a case worker. We looked through my financial records and I completed a multitude of forms. Medical assistance wouldn't solve all our problems but it would cover Bill's rehab when insurance stopped.

God, please help! You can do the impossible and heal Bill all the way. Surprise these medical people. Please!

The following day, Bill had an appointment with the neurologist from Bethesda whom I had not yet met.

Looking into Bill's face, the doctor spoke. "You're doing better. I'm encouraged by your improvement."

The doctor turned toward me. "I see he's on quite a few blood pressure medications. They might be dulling his cognitive functioning."

Thinking back, I realized Bill had seemed slower in thinking and activity since diagnosis with high blood pressure six years earlier.

"Do you think that being with dementia patients could deter Bill's improvement," I asked the doctor.

"Very possibly," he replied.

One more reinforcement in the case for moving Bill to fourth floor. Maybe.

After the appointment, Bill and I had lunch at an Indian restaurant he had remodeled right before his accident. We enjoyed Indian food and a reunion with the workers.

As we covered forty miles of the city, Bill read road signs. I was surprised by how well he remembered our metro's roads and landmarks.

This outing hinted of the ordinary life I longed for.

Where Next?

"IT LOOKS LIKE Bill may move to fourth floor tomorrow," said Bill's nurse.

"That would be wonderful!" My prayers were being answered. Maybe.

"Someone is leaving there today so there will be an opening." She frowned. "Our main concern, though, is whether he'll cooperate. He has been trying to remove his wander alert band. Last Friday, he walked out the front door."

"Yes, I heard about that. Is he getting any better?"

"I don't think he's tried it since, but there's no guarantee. When staff caught him and brought him back in, he cooperated without resistance."

"That's good." I sighed. "I hope this works out!" But something told me this might not happen.

"I'm scheduled to work on fourth tomorrow night. If he's there, I'll be sure to keep an eye on him."

Things were looking up.

The next morning Michelle, the social worker, called. "No decision has been made to move Bill to fourth floor. The daytime charge nurse doesn't advise it. She doesn't have confidence in his being able to handle it."

"Why?"

"Yesterday he walked off the unit twice. Then during the study today with the chaplain, he got up to leave two times. They can't interrupt what they're doing to redirect him back in," said Michelle.

"Can't they try it anyway? Bill's neurologist agreed that being with Alzheimer's patients wasn't helping," I pleaded.

"The fourth floor is busier with people coming and going. Also, the elevators are more accessible. He could escape easily and we would lose him." She paused and continued. "There is a vacancy but we don't think that this roommate would be a good one. Too belligerent. Bill needs to be in a more peaceful environment."

"Okay." Obviously I needed to trust their judgment in spite of my disappointment.

ಸಿ

July 4, Independence Day, I felt anything but free. When Bill lay unconscious in India, progress and problems were obvious and easy to explain. Now the needs were subtle. I didn't want to embarrass Bill by disclosing too much about his confusion nor did I want to bare my heart to hundreds of readers. I wrote to a selected "safe" group.

> Please bear with me as I share my heart. This morning in church, I got in touch again with my current delicate and weighty role. For 30+ years, we were a team. We made big decisions together. As each other's best friend, we shared our hearts, striving to understand the other's feelings. Though not perfect, our relationship strengthened both of us. Suddenly, things changed. Now I make decisions about and for my husband. Communication is extremely difficult. He knows that life is not normal, but is beset with chaos over even simple things. I struggle with guilt for having him at a nursing home, especially when he is frustrated.
>
> We are trusting God to bring him further than this. However, we must face the possibility of which we've been warned. Medical people remind us that Bill could stop

improving at any point. If he stops now, we can't postpone bringing him home indefinitely.

Please pray for wisdom and peace. Quite honestly, Mom and I would bear the greatest part of this load. It's overwhelming.

Thank you from the bottom of my heart for standing with us. I sure hope that I don't become a burden and wear out our friendships. One thing for sure is that I'm learning a lot about how to help others through the wonderful ways in which you partner with me.

Lying in bed, I flopped from side to side trying to relax. I sensed that God wanted to burn something into my heart. He wanted me to stop fretting and turn *everything* over with *thanksgiving* for His provision *before experiencing it*.

Lord, I need Your empowerment so I'm ready for anything. Bill's healing isn't happening according to my plans and my ways.

The red digits on the clock blazed 2:05 into the darkness.

I couldn't stop being Bill's advocate, making sure he had everything possible for wholeness.

If I really loved my husband, I would bring him home and not leave him at that place. Yet I still felt sick when I considered the thought. After being with Bill and hearing his accounts of the strange world within his brain, I welcomed returning home or work where conversations made sense. Now I understood why the social workers and others had advised me to take care of myself. This is the "long haul" they had warned me about.

Though it seemed right to wait for Bill's return home, I struggled with guilt. Was I hindering his improvement?

God, You created Bill. You also restore and re-create. I can't heal Bill. No one can make him well. It's by Your power, regardless of where he is.

Remembering that my sister, Lu, had worked with brain injury rehab, I emailed her the next day.

She replied that I needed to determine what actions would make a difference versus which ones were guilt-driven. She advised against bringing Bill home until he was ready. I would know when the time was right. Her letter lifted a huge load.

The maelstrom continued daily. Bill leaned toward John with a woeful, pleading expression and lowered his voice. "I must tell you that babies are being executed and their remains are cooked in the food. This is why I won't eat the food."

John and I exchanged looks. If Bill wouldn't listen to John, he wouldn't listen to anyone. John shook his head firmly. "Bill, I don't think you have to worry about that."

"Another thing that happened is that a man on the T.V. scolded me for praying and preaching." He sighed. "Please, help make these things right."

Bill's stories ranged from humorous to pathetic to bizarre. His roommate was using his stereo to bulldoze a place outside their room that was going to be a bathroom. A ninety-year-old woman was about to give birth.

Bill's *confabulations*, distortions of what was happening, seemed so real to him. I hated seeing him tormented by these. I suspected that dreams, incorrect perceptions of conversations, and T.V. blurred together in his mind. As time passed, he accumulated garbled stories.

Wondering if sleep medications caused the illusions, I talked to a nurse. She obtained permission from the doctor to try cutting back.

๛

Though the addled stories stopped, Bill didn't forget prior ones. Consequently, guilt plagued him about what he thought he had done wrong. No matter how hard I tried, I couldn't talk him into letting those issues go.

Bump on the Road

As July ended, Bill remained in the locked unit. His social worker advised us to gradually increase the length of home visits. She suggested that we take him to church and other places to participate in regular activities.

Friends planned a reunion for all who had been involved with Okontoe. For over 14 years, Bill had ministered with his dad to hundreds of people through this wilderness-based ministry.

We took Bill to the event, which was held at a nearby church. It began Friday night. Bill recognized people and remembered events we had shared with them. Many commented about Bill's favorable recovery.

Afterwards, Bill slept at home for the first time in six months. Saturday morning he made a pot of tea with minimal help from Mom. After breakfast, we returned to the reunion. He seemed energized by the love, affirmations and conversations. By the end of the day, he was exhausted and welcomed solitude.

Sunday morning, he awakened after six hours of sleep and asked about the day's plans. We attended church. Though he strained to understand everything, he fit into the familiar routine. That afternoon he found ice cream in the freezer and dished up two bowlfuls, one for me and one for himself.

Bill's brother Don and his family were back in the States and came for lunch on Monday. The brothers stood guard over burgers and hotdogs on the grill. Bill found the long-handled utensils and dug out a pan for cooked meat. This was noteworthy because it was *normal*.

After lunch, Bill checked the time. "I think I should go back to Tr...Trev...ella."

※

On Tuesday, we had another family meeting. Michelle talked with Bill beforehand.

"Bill and I had a good meeting." She handed me a sheet. "This is what I gave to Bill. His thinking was clear and he understood."

"That's good," I replied, grateful for a good report.

"He seems analytical," she said.

"Does this have to do with the amount of education and intelligence before brain injury?"

"I'm sure it's an advantage." She pulled a sheet from her file. "Yes, I see here that he got a Master of Divinity after a B.A. He's a well-educated man."

The meeting's outcome wasn't what I had expected. The staff reiterated their concerns about moving Bill to fourth floor. Because of their own issues, other residents would not tolerate his tendency to interrupt, preach, or pray for them. Emotionally, it would be hard for Bill. They felt that a temporary move wasn't worth the stress it would cause him.

Trevilla's therapy program couldn't do much more for him, and insurance coverage for residential care would end soon. The best option was not a group home, but ours.

Home. Now this felt right. Though Bill still talked about erroneous incidents, he wasn't generating new ones.

Michele arranged for us to meet with a county worker and public health nurse for discussing our options. All agreed that someone needed to be with Bill all the time. We discussed whether or not we needed an alarm system to alert us if he tried to escape. So far he hadn't shown any tendencies to sneak out. Instead, he routinely locked the door after making sure everyone was inside.

Courage Center could provide further rehab and adult day care some days. We needed to begin the application process immediately since it tended to take a few weeks.

Evaluations and interviews consumed the next week, resulting in Bill's certification as *disabled*. This qualified him for medical assistance which would pay for further rehabilitation and medically related transportation. Though relieved, I wondered if my husband would bear the *disabled* label for the rest of his life.

Would life seem so normal that he would try to drive one of the cars? If so, how would we stop him? We would hide our car keys and hope he didn't dig for them. Would he accept my explanations without thinking I was trying to control him?

Grace. It's meaning was now personal, not theoretical. Grace: the subtle, stabilizing source of peace helping me persevere, the glue holding me together. Grace had dissolved the terror. Life went on and wasn't out of control. *God is in control and I can rest in that.* Prayers of people worldwide carried me.

I reflected on a recent sermon about keys. As we turn in our keys to Jesus, He gives us new ones. Our keys are the old ways of doing things which worked in the past. *I have sure been turning in lots of keys lately!* Our conditions would give way to the glory of God. How could Bill's outcome be anything but good if he was to be a demonstration of God's glory?

On July 27, I wrote in my journal:

> I must take one step at a time, trusting that God's plan is good. His plan shapes us into His image. Remembering this helped me settle into a peaceful place, to tame the wild animal thoughts that ran me out of bed this morning.
>
> Lord, as I walk through this day, I trust You to lead me step by step. You will work out the kinks as I let You. There are too many things to think about without Your help. I'm learning to find Your will instead of depending upon Bill. Lord, please help Bill to hear You again instead of the mixed-up voices of his weakened condition.

‌‌‌

Lined with blooming plants, paved paths wound around grassy slopes. Mom and I parked in a lot behind the large three-story brick structure built into the side of a hill. Following a path to Courage Center's main entrance, we walked past a children's play area. Extended roof vans lined up along the curb to drop off or pick up passengers. I watched a lift lower a man seated in a wheelchair.

At the glassed in entrance, we slowed behind a woman using a walker. Inside we approached a desk in front of a glass wall through which we could see an Olympic-sized swimming pool. One side of the pool area sloped into the water.

"May I help you?" asked the receptionist also sitting in a wheelchair.

"Yes, we're here to tour the center and meet with someone in the Adult Day Program."

"Tim will be with you shortly. He'll take you up there."

We waited in a spacious foyer with a mezzanine flanked by huge plants. The facility resembled a college campus, a place of dignity. *Lord, let this work out please!*

A man in a motorized chair approached. His pant legs were folded under at hip level because he had no legs. With a short stub for an arm, he drove himself toward us smiling.

"Hello. I'm Tim. Follow me. We'll take these elevators to second floor."

He led us throughout the building describing Courage Center's offerings in occupational therapy, career development, exercise, residential care, community reintegration, driver's training and adult day care. "Our mission is to empower people with physical disabilities to reach their full potential in every aspect of life."

"That's wonderful." I responded.

"Yes, our vision is that all will live, work, learn and play in a community based on abilities, not disabilities."

If anyone could assist Bill back to a full, satisfying life, Courage Center could.

Bump on the Road

Tim introduced us to the head of Adult Day Care and left. She led us into her office where we talked about Bill's situation. She said that openings were limited but, if their program was a good fit, they would provide more days as spots opened up.

We left hopeful, impressed, and hopeful that this wouldn't be another "no."

The last weekend of July, I picked up Bill and we headed north for church family camp. Recognizing the route from previous trips, he told me where to turn.

He labored to follow group conversations and to understand what was happening next. Though he enjoyed being with friends, he tired quickly. Often, he withdrew for a nap. Now I functioned as an extrovert and he an introvert, opposite to our pre-accident styles. I craved logical, intelligent discussions.

After the weekend at camp, I took Bill back to Trevilla. This was beginning to feel unnecessary. However, I was thankful for time to organize our home.

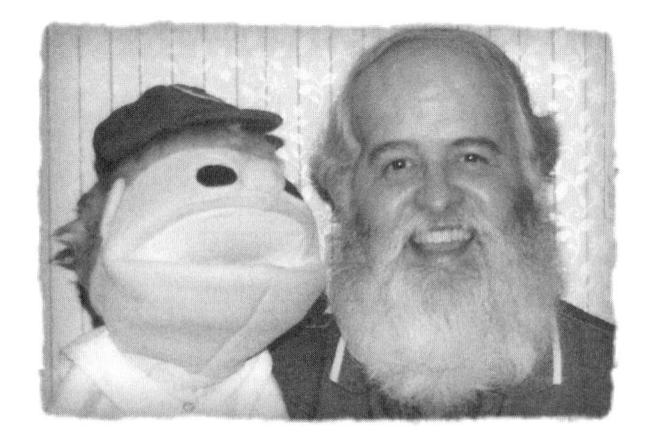

Home at Last

"GUESS WE'D BETTER tackle the basement," I said as we finished supper.

"Can I help?" asked Mom as she loaded the dishwasher.

"I think we can manage. Your doing dishes is a big help."

Jody and I descended to the bowels of our house and stared at the leftovers from Bill's last project.

"How on earth are we going to do this?" Jody groaned.

"I guess we'll have to try to sort it into categories and throw out what's obviously trash," I said.

"I sure hope Dad can find his stuff. Do you think he'll ever do this kind of project again?"

"I don't know." I picked up a board which was the remains of a scalloped archway he had made for an Indian restaurant. "He sure did a top-notch job. Spent hours figuring out the design. It was rather complicated."

"Do we need to save that piece?" she asked.

"Might be a good idea in case they ask him to do another one. Could use it as a pattern."

Jody went into the adjacent storage room and returned. "What do you think about moving all the boxes of books in here? Then we could use the shelves in his work area for his carpentry stuff."

"Good idea. If we organize logically, he can at least find things. Who knows if he'd remember where things were."

"Or what he had."

Bump on the Road

"At least it will be more orderly and that should help." I envisioned giving Bill a tour of his work area, wondering if he would be aware enough to be offended with our meddling. "He's supposed to have a clutter-free environment. Hopefully, this helps."

Three hours later, the floor was visible at last.

Friday, August 6, closed one chapter and began another. I finished work early and headed to Trevilla one last time.

Had we known how long it would take for Bill to return home, would we have boarded that flight to Delhi in January?

Skirting roadwork on Highway 100, I wondered how much longer the reconstruction of Bill would require. His physical detour had changed him to a child. Or an old man. How would he feel about his mother, wife, and daughter telling him what he could and couldn't do? Would he expect to re-enter his former independence?

I needed God's help, no matter what. Total recovery would be a miracle, but so would living with a disabled spouse "till death do us part."

How would Bill fill his days? Qualms remained but I knew it was time for Bill to return home to stay.

I toted two large suitcases into Trevilla. A nursing assistant helped pack and load Bill's things onto a cart. Then the charge nurse brought me a stack of papers to sign.

"This is the first time we have discharged someone to go *home* from this unit." With the back of her hand, the nurse brushed away tears. "He is doing so well, and should do fine in familiar surroundings."

"I agree." No more worries about the influence of confused companions.

"Come back and visit, okay Bill?" The nurse shook Bill's hand.

At home, the aroma of roast beef, potatoes and carrots met us. Mom set the table as I pulled 3-bean salad and applesauce from the fridge. It didn't take long to discover a new quandary.

Home at Last

Bill ate as though each meal was his last opportunity. I resorted to rescuing serving dishes from Bill's reach until I knew everyone else was finished. Then I put away leftovers immediately.

※

Our lives, which had been like divergent streams, finally started flowing together. Familiar surroundings triggered appropriate responses like letting the dog out, setting the table, making juice, discussing plans for the day, playing CDs, and more.

We had traveled through the dark, winter days of our commitment "in sickness and in health ... as long as we both shall live." Now spring was overcoming a long winter. My husband's disinterest and emotional flatness were gone. The brain injury had not stolen Bill's kind, compassionate personality.

Bill frequently brought up his ministry, the future, and what he would do. I appreciated his thinking ahead but wondered how much he could do now. Most of his previous work had required more problem-solving skills than he presently had.

How would I be his "helpmeet" now? I needed to be sensitive to when and how to gradually let go. It was a strange season of role reversal. He often didn't grasp why this was necessary, and I struggled to help him understand.

As he improved, he grew increasingly aware. Along with that, he felt responsible over his "departments."

With five or more at our table some days, dinner conversations resembled rapidly popping popcorn. He struggled to keep abreast of the interchange. He either asked me to repeat or dozed. He did best when he could initiate conversation, expressing his own thoughts. Even so, he had moments of *aphasia* – struggling to remember the word he wanted to use. "So Bill, are you really going to pack your swimming *pool* in your gym bag and you're taking your lunch in a *suitcase*?"

Bump on the Road

After dinner one evening, I talked Bill into going for a walk with me. As we chatted about various things, I realized his auditory perception was improving. As if he had heard my thoughts, he said, "I have been having difficulty understanding conversations the past couple of days. Especially when there's a lot going on."

"Really?" I replied. "I was thinking that you're doing better. You're understanding more now than when you first came home."

"Oh?" He didn't sound convinced.

I wondered if his awareness of this problem marked a step forward, a sign that he was getting better.

"I need to talk to you about something else, too. I feel badly about what happened at Tre... Trevla..."

"What is it?" I hoped it wasn't the same old misperception.

"It was that time that the woman from down the hall..." His discourse trailed off and didn't make sense.

"Bill, we've talked about this before. I really don't think that happened. I'm sure you dreamed it. You had crazy dreams when you were on medication to help you sleep."

Would I ever convince him that these things didn't happen?

"No, you don't understand. I need to make things right."

"Bill, honest, you didn't do anything wrong!" I stopped, grabbed his hand and looked him in the eye. "You were with people who were confused. More confused than you were. They were saying wacky things. Your perception was goofy and so was theirs."

"But ..."

I stomped my foot. "Please. Believe me! I don't want to see you agonizing over this any longer!" We trudged the remaining half block home.

As we entered the back door, Mom asked, "Did you have a pleasant walk?"

"I guess so," Bill replied.

"What's wrong, Dad?" Jody asked.

I didn't give him a chance to respond. "Oh, he's still convinced that certain things occurred at Trevilla that didn't."

"Dad." Jody stood in front of him and looked him in the eye. "Mom's right. Those things didn't happen. Please believe us!"

"Honey," Mom chimed in, "these thoughts are harassing you. Please let it go! It's stealing your joy and…" She slapped the counter. "I won't have it!" When the stack of plates rattled, she flinched with embarrassment over her mild outburst.

"Me neither! I'm tired of you being upset over these things that aren't true," I declared. Pouring on more drama, I pled, "Don't you believe us? We're not lying to you! Why would we? We love you and want you to be happy."

Bill's countenance dropped another six inches. "You don't understand…"

"I don't want to talk about it anymore." I turned and stormed out of the room.

Bill sauntered into the living room, sat in the green recliner and dozed off.

I returned to the kitchen and cried with Mom and Jody.

An invitation came in the mail from Bethesda:
BETHESDA ALUMNI PICNIC
FRIDAY, SEPTEMBER 10, 1999
FAMILY WELCOME, TOO

Eager to show Bethesda staff how well Bill was doing, I talked my husband into attending. As I drove toward downtown St. Paul, Bill challenged, "Why are we going this way?"

"This is how we get to Bethesda!"

He frowned.

As the state capitol came into view, I exited the freeway.

"Where are we going?" Bill quizzed again.

"We're going to Bethesda to the picnic."

"Oh, is it here?"

"Yes, this is Bethesda right here." *Trust me, would you?*

I found a parking spot two blocks away. I hopped out as he inched his way slowly from the passenger seat. Straightening his cap, he looked across the street. "That's the state capitol!"

"You don't remember seeing the capitol from your floor?" I recalled pointing it out to him but wondering if he understood.

"Umm, I guess I remember seeing it out the window. I thought I was somewhere south. By the Iowa border."

Taking his hand, I pulled him along the sidewalk toward Bethesda's main entrance. People milled around and sat in groups at long tables, eating hotdogs, chips, and cake. We helped ourselves and sat by a man and woman.

Glancing around I searched for familiar faces. I didn't recognize any former patients though I saw familiar staff. They commented about how well Bill was doing. I agreed.

We chatted with others about head injury and recovery. Their stories uplifted me.

"Let's go upstairs to see where you were," I said.

"I don't feel the need to."

Convinced that seeing his former ward would help Bill connect the dots, I was determined. I wanted him to understand his process of recovery and why he still had limitations. "I'd like to go up there and I think it would be encouraging for them to see how well you are doing now." I took him by the hand and led him along as a mother does with a reluctant child. He complied. We went through the double door entry, down a hall, around a corner, up the elevator to the all-too-familiar set of locked doors.

"Where are we?" he asked.

"This is where you stayed while you were here."

Glancing to the left, he said, "I remember this room. That's where Deanna gave us an organ concert. That was beautiful! She even knew how to play 'Twinkle Twinkle Little Star.' Amazing!"

"Yes, that's right," I said as I rang the doorbell.

A nurse came from within. Cracking it open a few inches, she asked, "May I help you?"

"Yes," I replied. "This is Bill Barr. He was a patient in this unit last spring. We came for the alumni picnic and I wanted to show him where he had been."

"Come on in."

As we entered the TV area, the same in-your-face patient greeted us. *What sort of insurance allowed him to be here so long?* As before, a nurse gently redirected him.

"Hello Bill! Did you come to visit?"

"Yes." Straining to read the tag dangling from a strap around her neck, he asked, "I'm sorry, I don't remember your name."

"I'm Christy. Do you remember me? I took care of you while you were here."

"Yes, I remember you... Christy. Right?"

Nodding in reply, she asked, "So where are you now?"

"I am living at home now. I'm going to Courage Center for some more treatment there."

Taking Bill's hand, I led him toward his former room. "Do you remember this room, Bill?"

"I think so." He walked closer.

I pulled him back. "It's someone else's room now."

"Okay, let's go home." Bill turned around and headed toward the door.

Christy extended her hand. "It was good to see you, Bill."

"Thank you, and your name is?" He read her tag and beamed. "Christy."

Thanking God for freedom from the locked unit, I led Bill back to the car. The only markers we wore were name tags from the alumni picnic in the courtyard. Four months ago, I regretted that Bill had to leave that place. Now I was thankful that he could.

Courage

September 13, 1999 Journal:

Lord, I'm overwhelmed and burnt out. Please help me have "mini vacations." Help us order our lives. Disorder gets to Bill, but we have a hard time getting organized. Revelation 7:17 promises that the the Lord will comfort me, wiping away my tears. I need it!

When I showered yesterday, Bill stood outside the clouded shower door. When I shut off the shower briefly, he opened the door to hand me a towel. His sweet gesture illustrated his life. He stands on the edge, looking in and trying to understand. The form is there but indistinct like the steamed glass divider between us.

I'm desperate for daily wisdom and grace, Lord. With the pressures and busyness, I get irritated explaining and repeating everything multiple times. It's easier to say nothing and keep thoughts inside. Lord, I don't want to cut myself off.

Thank You, Lord, that he can go to Courage Center three days a week now. He seems to enjoy it and we get a break. Since he has therapy two of those days, I only have to drive him once a week. It seems like nothing after commuting that distance daily for six months. I'm so glad the public health nurse got through to him about the tormenting memories from Trevilla. He finally seemed convinced that those crazy things didn't happen. Hallelujah. We're making progress. I must focus on the positive.

"I had a good talk with Ed today," reported Bill when he arrived home from Courage Center.

"What did you talk about?" I asked.

"I told him that I want to get back into work and I would like to drive again. He said that they could give me a driving assessment and that I might be able to get vocational counseling later."

"That's good." I was grateful someone else could manage these questions for now. I couldn't picture Bill driving. Not yet, anyway.

The driving evaluation was scheduled for September 20.

When he arrived home that day, I asked, "How did the test go?"

"Different."

"In what way?"

"It was this big board with lights. I had to push buttons when the lights flashed as fast as I could. It was really frustrating!"

"It sounds like they were testing your reaction time."

"It didn't make any sense to me." He sighed. "My therapist sent this bucket home with me today." Something rattled when he set the five-quart ice cream container on the table. "She wants me to work on this stuff at home."

"That sounds good! Can I see it?" I was all for anything that would help Bill regain former competencies.

"Yeah, go ahead." His enthusiasm didn't match mine.

Opening it, I saw little Ziploc bags containing small things such as buttons, paper clips, and pins along with instruction for what to do with the items. "This looks like it will help your manual dexterity."

"Yeah, but I don't know why I need it."

He fumbled with the lid until it snapped on and stashed the bucket in a corner where it remained.

One Wednesday on the way to Courage Center we rode in silence interrupted occasionally by Bill's "back seat driving." Unforeseen distractions that morning had aborted my plan to have a quiet time.

Bump on the Road

I prayed silently as I drove. Then I felt that I was supposed to talk to Bill about what was bothering me.

"Bill, would you pray with me about something?"

"Sure, what's that?"

"I'm starting a women's group tonight at church, but the marriage group will probably attract all the women." I paused, letting my words sink into his brain. "Last time I led a group at the same time as another person. She had a big group and I had one woman. I don't want to go to church on Wednesday nights for just one or two people."

Bill cleared his throat. "Lord, I pray for Cheryl that you would bless her and give her peace. I pray that You would bring those You want to have in her Bible study. Lord, I ask that You would surprise her and bless her with a really good group and that lots of people would come! Thank You, Lord!"

I exhaled. "Thanks!" A heavy load lifted. "That helped a lot." Maybe I was getting my closest confidant and friend back, after all.

As it turned out, my classroom filled with a delightful group of women.

Sun light filtered through the maple branches outside, now that some leaves had fallen. Bill was in the kitchen making coffee. Clad in my favorite flannel pajamas, I sat in bed with pillows wedged behind me as I wrote.

October 9, 1999 Journal:

Lying in bed this morning, a thought surfaced. "Depression comes from non-acceptance of losing control of one's life." If this is the case, the best cure for depression is giving control to God, letting Him have it. He should be in charge because He is the Potter and we are the clay. It's impossible for us to see the whole picture and our part in God's plan. He allows and causes what He wills for a much bigger purpose. I need to remember this when discouraged.

Why aren't I more grateful that Bill is doing as well as he is? The crisis is past, but the highs of marked improvements are marred by Bill's incompleteness. Talking to Bill requires so much effort. I often shout as though he were deaf, but it doesn't help. He looks so sad as he implores me to not yell at him.

Realignment of our roles challenges both of us. As he's able to handle more, I struggle to release. Letting him own a little responsibility is scary.

Our harmonious marriage has become discordant. *How can I lovingly and respectfully relate to a spouse who is now like a thirteen year old?* I wonder if he feels trapped by three and, sometimes, four mothers—me, Jody, Mom, and Joy when she's here.

When I woke up the other day, Bill was eating leftover pizza as dessert to a peanut butter sandwich. Last night, after sleeping two hours, he munched a chocolate donut. His weight has reached an all time high. Has he lost his ability to discern when he's full? Doesn't he notice indigestion?

That morning's devotional reading about raisins arrested my heart. Choice grapes are bathed in hot water; dehydrated twenty-four hours in carefully established warmth; gently washed in warm water, and then packaged so they become moist and tasty.

Did God choose us and allow this to happen because we were choice?

Raisins serve a purpose. Since they are preserved, they are ideal for camping trips, kids' lunches, and keeping on hand for emergencies. They endure much more than fresh grapes. Maybe that's why God wants to make us into raisins.

During the peak of crisis, I didn't complain about small stuff. I was busy with important issues and decisions. But now? I prayed earlier that this trial would not be wasted by my slipping back into old ways. Would I look at Bill's deficits or at his progress? Yes, Bill's deficiencies were part of life now. Life had changed. *I must hang onto a good attitude to survive whatever comes.*

As Moses led the Israelites out of Egypt thousands of years ago, they grumbled on the heels of remarkable victories. Though they had just miraculously marched through the Red Sea, they complained because they didn't have water to drink. Fear displaced the joy of freedom from Egypt's captivity.

Perseverance in the heat of refinement would make me a better person–a raisin, suitable for hardship conditions!

Lord, help me to be patient. Give me grace for Bill's disability.

༄

Early November on a Sunday eve, I sat on the living room floor amongst piles of pictures. Memories.

I turned toward Bill who lounged above me in the recliner. "Bill, here's a picture of the doctor and nurse with you on the airplane."

"Can I see it?"

I handed the picture to him.

After studying it, he handed it back. "Were they with me the whole time?"

"They sat across the aisle from you. One slept while the other took care of you."

"What did they need to do for me?"

"They fed you through the tube in your nose every two hours."

"A tube through my nose?"

"Yes, it went in through your nose and down to your stomach. You weren't awake enough to eat."

"Where did they get the food?"

"They brought it with them."

"What was it?"

"One time the nurse said it was tomato soup."

"Tomato soup?"

He paused. "Did they feed me tomato soup here, too?"

"No. When you were in ICU the nurse showed me a can of what they gave you. The little can had all kinds of ingredients. Even beef." I made a 4" deep "C" with my hand to indicate its size.

"Humph! So I had beef in ICU?" he chuckled.

"Here are the nurses and doctors in India."

Then I handed him a photo that showed hundreds of staples arching across the right side of his head. "This is at North Memorial right before the stitches were removed."

He pointed at another picture. "Who's that?"

"That's how you looked before they put in the bone piece. See how your head was indented?"

"Uh huh," he replied.

"The swelling had gone down. Since the bone wasn't there, it looked indented. We were relieved when they replaced the bone! It was dangerous having your brain exposed like that. Besides, you look better!"

He pointed to the scar on his forehead. "This is where they put me back together."

I nodded.

"Here's a picture of your farewell at Bethesda. See, you were starting to connect with others by then."

He nodded as he studied a picture of himself waving and smiling with a group of nurses.

"Here are some pictures from our trip before your accident. Do you remember these people?"

He studied the faces. "I think so."

I held up a picture of Scott and Anita's family. "Do you remember visiting these friends?"

He thought for a minute and nodded. "Yes, our friends."

Bump on the Road

Memories were returning in chunks. I remembered Dr. Harlow saying that Bill would remember India but not being in North Memorial. At the time his statement was a ray of hope. Now it was reality.

Then I showed him a picture of Brother Kaushal visiting Bill at Bethesda.

Bill smiled. "It was good to see Brother Kaushal again."

"Yes, he came to visit when he was in the States. He was very concerned about you and I'm glad he could see you when you were doing better."

Reaching for another picture, Bill said, "I remember those big pictures on the wall. Who made those?"

"It was Deb from church."

"Those pictures were awesome! Maybe we can put them up somewhere."

"Uh huh." I couldn't imagine what room to decorate with two two-foot by six-foot drawings done on brown wrapping paper. "What else do you remember about being at Bethesda?"

"I needed a shower before that surgery was done, but they wouldn't let me have one until I finally insisted upon it. They never did do the surgery." He chuckled humorlessly. "But they came into my room and simply yanked out the tube in my stomach. They didn't even tell me they were doing it!"

"No, they told you. Jody was there and she said they asked you if they could remove it and you agreed. They were so happy that you let them do it."

He shook his head. "They never did do that surgery that they were supposed to come and get me for."

"That was to remove your feeding tube and they did it in your room! They didn't have to take you out for it."

"It was mysterious." He chuckled dryly. "I didn't want to eat that recycled meat they kept giving me there."

"Do you remember anything else about Bethesda?" I asked.

"The children's choir. They were glorious! But they kept the door locked and wouldn't let me go back and hear them again."

"We talked about that already." I felt as though I were talking to a brick wall.

Bill started looking sleepy as though his processor was overloaded. What began as a good conversation was plummeting toward frustration for both of us. I put away the pictures and went into the kitchen where Jody was studying her anatomy books. She looked up and we exchanged bitter sweet looks.

November 15, 1999 Journal

Life is like riding on an Indian bus, standing with knees slightly flexed to absorb bumps in the road. We can't get there any faster by forcing our way, like when the tree was on the road blocking traffic. We looked for an out, but there wasn't one. Sometimes life comes to a standstill like that. We just need to wait and trust that we'll get through, as we eventually did on that Indian road. We'll get through this, too. We're settling into a different pace.

We weren't done leaning on God. I needed grace if Bill remained as he was now, but I also needed to press on in faith, believing God for further healing. Bill seemed discouraged and I suspected that he thought I wanted to be in charge.

God, Your Word says that You are faithful to complete what You've begun in us.

I remembered what I had seen through our kitchen window on Thanksgiving Day. Long after everything else had succumbed to frost and cooler temps, late blooming flowers stood within a circle of snow. Against all odds, hope presses through like those flowers.

Pre-accident, Bill usually respected my suggestions. Now it was different. I had to decide which battles to choose. Would he

Bump on the Road

put himself or others in danger by making a poor choice? It was time to back off as much as I could.

I wondered if Bill felt threatened to the core of his identity. Daily his losses scowled at him. He couldn't drive where and when he wanted to go. He had no job. Day in and day out, others told him what to do. Though we weren't in crisis mode now, different struggles consumed us.

I thought about how we are clay in the potter's hand. God shapes us according to His design. In pottery class, we "wedged" the clay to remove bubbles. We sliced the clay lump with a taut wire stretched above the table, then flung it onto the table several times. Removing air pockets kept our pottery from cracking in the hot kiln.

God desires to remove the air bubbles from our lives. If we resist, the process is more difficult. Circumstances like Bill's accident wedge the clay. I realized that God would rather not allow hardships, but sometimes there's no other way.

As a young woman I had feared yielding to God because of what He might require. Now I realized that, in releasing control to Him, He enables me to travel the rugged road.

The final year of the twentieth century had brought the greatest test of our lives. Yet I finished the year with stronger confidence in God's grace and faithfulness. Along with Bill's recovery and return home, we celebrated new life. Both of our sons had new babies. We entered a new century with five grandchildren. "Bompa" was alive and able to enjoy his grandbabies.

A New Year

JANUARY 4, Bill had an appointment with the neuropsychologist in the heart of downtown St. Paul. Near the crossover of two interstate freeways, I exited onto a grid of one-way streets. The two-inch thick map book was on Bill's lap as he attempted to navigate.

I tightened my grip on the steering wheel. We were running late. Again. Last time they had warned us that, if we were more than fifteen minutes late, we would lose our appointment time and need to reschedule.

We rounded a corner and there it was. *Thank goodness!* I pulled into the parking ramp and yanked a card from the ticket dispensing device.

"I don't see why we have to pay for parking to see a doctor!" I complained.

"What did you say?" asked Bill.

"Never mind. I wonder…."

"What?"

"Bill, maybe I should let you out here at the door so I can find a spot."

"No, let's stick together. I don't know where to go."

"Okay. But we've got to hurry!" How could I get my husband to move faster? "We can't be late or else we'll miss our appointment."

"I know, I know. Don't be mad at me!"

Three layers up, I finally found a parking spot.

Bump on the Road

"This is too small," said Bill. "You're going to scrape that other car."

"No, I'm not. There's plenty of room!"

I parked, bounded out, and charged around to his side. "Come on! We can't be late!" I wished I could grab him and carry him as I had with our kids.

Slowly my frustrated hubby extricated himself. "I'm coming!"

When he was out, I grabbed him by the hand and pulled him to the door, down the hall, to an elevator, through a skyway over the street below, down another hall to another elevator which we rode to ground level. There we hiked down another hallway to the check-in desk.

"Hi," I huffed and puffed. "This is Bill Barr. He's here for an appointment."

"Okay, please take a seat and fill out these forms." The receptionist handed me a clipboard with forms and motioned to the chairs lining the hallway across from her.

I took the clipboard, exhaled, and nudged Bill toward two empty chairs together. As I started to sit, Bill said that he needed to find the bathroom. "Well, all right. If you *have* to go right now."

"I'll be right back." He frowned.

"Okay but hurry!"

With hat in hand and coat still on, he ambled back down the hallway as I hurriedly filled out the forms.

Bill returned and signed the forms. Whew, we made it!

We waited as others were called in. I checked my watch. An hour had passed since our appointment time. I went to the receptionist to make sure we hadn't missed our appointment.

"The doctor is running late because he was called out for an emergency."

Another fifteen minutes, then it was our turn.

Bill chatted easily with the doctor, answering a few questions.

"I see a twinkle in your eye and that your sense of humor is returning," said the doctor. "Your articulation has improved, even since the last time you were here two months ago. You seem to be doing very well, Bill. I'm glad to see that. I think we can gradually cut back on antidepressants and take you off them eventually."

Bill smiled. "That's good."

We left his office with improved moods.

"Our friend, James, is in Regions Hospital," I said. "He had surgery yesterday. Would you like to go see him while we're in the area?"

"Sure," Bill replied.

Thanks to the thick map book, we found Regions Hospital and parked in another ramp. Again, I grabbed Bill's hand and dragged him down hallways, up and down elevators to find our friend.

We found James, and his wife. Bill fell naturally into the pastoral role. He greeted James, talked briefly, listened to James' story of ending up in the hospital, prayed for the couple, and said, "We need to go now."

"Thanks so much for coming up to see me!" James grabbed Bill's hand. "Thank you, Lord." James closed his eyes and smiled.

I remembered when James sat by Bill at North Memorial Hospital. A look of despair had lingered on James' face as Bill lay expressionless next to him.

∞

Driving home one blizzardy night, I couldn't see the road. Snow and ice pack covered the lines on the freeway. I followed the tail lights ahead of me, hoping the vehicle didn't inadvertently lead me into a ditch.

Then I saw a snow plow ahead. Did its driver know where the road edges were? How do they know where to plow, espe-

Bump on the Road

cially if the road is unfamiliar and curvy? Signs above the highway were our only guides.

I was relieved to reach my exit safely.

This reminded me of our uncertain future. Though much better, Bill hadn't caught up to what he used to be. How would his life unfold now? Hope for a 100% recovery waned. Even before brain injury, we had struggled to understand God's purposes for us. We had been headed in a direction that now seemed impossible. What was hard before was now unimaginable. Since Plan A isn't happening, what's Plan B?

Lord, help! Please show us road markers through the storm so we don't slide into the ditch!

My husband wanted and needed significance and purpose. It seemed that his strengths and abilities had been stripped away. Instead of planning his next trip overseas, he was figuring out who would take him a half mile to the local hardware store. Rather than solving our technical and electronic problems, he now asked how to put in a movie. He who had interpreted medical jargon for others was now challenged to organize his medications.

How could we help him understand his condition without devastating him? Can he grasp the outpouring of love so he could simply rest in the blessing?

Even though Bill struggled with usefulness, I couldn't persuade him to help with simple things around the house. It was as though he was stuck in quicksand. Whenever I asked him to do something, he usually said, "It's a possibility."

I felt like screaming. Why couldn't he simply say, *yes*?

At times he did what I asked after analyzing the process. Then he slowly ambled into action, taking several detours along the way. Much later, he finished.

Desiring objective help, I arranged a meeting with Pastor Gordy and Jana at their home.

A New Year

A fire crackled in the fireplace as Jana served tea from the coffee table between us. Bill talked of wanting to find ministry again. I described my frustrations about his reluctance to help at home.

"I see four things for you to work on," began our pastor. "Both of you are in a grief process, dealing with losses even though you did not lose your life, Bill. Whenever there is a loss, there are adjustments to be made regardless of whether the loss is temporary or permanent." He paused to sip tea. "I would like you to make a list of your losses, ask what this means to you, give them to the Lord, and ask for His comfort."

I hadn't thought of it that way, but his words rang true.

"What should I do about ministry?" Bill asked.

"Your value is not based on what you *do* in ministry. You are valuable just because of who you are as a child of God. He loves you and so do we. What you do doesn't give you value but rather who you *are* as His beloved child."

Bill nodded.

"One effect of your accident is difficulty in hearing. Before your accident you had excellent listening skills. Now you need to redevelop those, and you can." Pastor hesitated, giving Bill a chance to grasp his words. "Finally, trust that those around you have your best interests in mind. You are surrounded by people who love you and want the best for you." He paused. "Does this make sense?"

"Yes, I think so."

"Remember reading about King Nebuchadnezzar, in the Old Testament?" asked Pastor Gordy. "He had lost his mind. Of course, his situation was different. However, when he looked to God and called out to Him, his mind was restored. I believe that, as you call upon God, He will help you and restore your mind. Recovery and restoration are gifts from God."

Lord, please awaken Bill's brain cells so he will seek You for deliverance from the tyranny of his confused mind!

Leaving Pastor's home, I felt pounds lighter.

Bump on the Road

Bill was in his basement office playing Free Cell on the computer as I cooked supper. Jody emerged from a pile of books on the living room floor where she was studying. She stretched her legs and rubbed her back. "Aargh. Had to get up and move around a bit." She grabbed a tomato slice from the salad I was making.

"I saw that," I bantered.

"You know how I've been longing for Dad's counsel and advice about my marrying Ben? I've struggled with wondering if I was doing the right thing because of missions and all. I decided to share my heart with Dad and come right out and ask what he thought."

"What did he say?"

"He said my spirit knows that it is right. That was the confirmation I needed. It's been evident all along that Dad's spirit was not damaged. Now I have peace about marrying Ben."

"Good." I was relieved too.

Jody snitched a pepper chunk from the cutting board. "All my life I've dreamed of Dad doing my wedding, but now ... do you think he's able to do it?"

"I think so. Part of it, at least. Maybe Pastor Gordy could work with him," I answered.

"I was thinking that, too." She sighed longingly. "I don't know if he could do it by himself. You know what I mean?"

"Yeah. It's hard to know what would kick in." I pulled some salad tongs from the drawer. "He's done many weddings but ..."

"He seems to be getting better, and it's another six months away. I'd really like for him to do it even though it wouldn't be the same as it would have been before. We meet with Pastor Gordy on Thursday so we'll talk to him and see what he thinks."

A New Year

After their appointment with Pastor Gordy on Thursday, Ben joined us for supper. "How was your appointment with Pastor Gordy today?" asked Bill.

"Good. We took the pre-marriage evaluation last week and today we went over the results," said Jody. "Pastor said things look good." She smiled at Ben.

"Yep. We passed the test." He chuckled and drew Jody close.

"Dad, we would like to have you help do the ceremony. Would you like to do it?"

"Yes." Bill's eyes twinkled. "I would be honored."

"Pastor Gordy said he would help. Do you think you could come up with a message?" Jody asked.

"Sure. I've done those many times," said Bill.

I hoped he wasn't overconfident.

Jody glanced at Ben and he nodded. She swallowed and said, "We talked about getting married in July. Probably the eighth."

My daughter was leaving the nest in a few months. Gulp. Bill asked Jody to pass the bread. Then he began describing our wedding and how I had finished college after we were married.

"I'll keep going to school and get my degree. With Ben working, we figured out that we can swing it financially."

Bill paused a half second so Jody continued, "We talked to Ben's parents about having an outdoor wedding at their place."

"Did you know that's a Barr-girl tradition?" said Bill. "We had three weddings outside at Okontoe." Bill described the weddings of his three sisters.

"It was lots of work but did reduce the cost," I said.

"Because we don't have a lawn yet," said Ben. "we told Dad and Mom that we would plant grass."

"We'll have that as the front with the chairs facing the small grove of trees," said Jody.

I remembered standing in the unfinished log house with Marilee as she described the layout. At the time, nine of them crammed into a mobile home on the property temporarily. Ben shared a dresser with three brothers, having one drawer as his own. I don't know how they survived. Now, at last, they were finally spreading out in the almost finished house.

It would be a lovely rural setting. A half-mile-long dirt driveway wrapped around a corn field with woods on the other side.

Jody turned toward me, hesitating briefly. "Mom, do you suppose you could make my wedding dress?"

"I'd be honored to."

"I'm getting an idea but want to try on some dresses at bridal shops." She grinned at her fiance.

He wiggled his brows in reply.

JOURNAL January 25, 2000

I'm learning through experience, not just intellectually Through this trial, I'm discovering God's help, wisdom and love. How would I comprehend these attributes of God if I didn't need help? I had known that I needed to lean on God more and less on Bill, but knowing and doing are vastly different. Now I'm pressed to lean on God since I can't lean on Bill anymore. Good is coming from this. I hope I don't regress to the narrow, self-centered person that I was before.

Later that day, Bill and I sat with Joel and Bridget at their house. I looked at my watch. "You know what I just realized?" I said. "A year ago right now, Bill had his accident. It was January 26 at 8:00 a.m. there but it was still January 25 here."

"That's right!" said Bridget.

Joel grimaced. "I'll never forget that night!"

"Me neither!" Bridget snuggled closer to Joel. "We were sound asleep when the phone rang."

"It was awful! Peter telling us that Dad was in a bad accident. Neither of us slept after that. I didn't work the next day. Couldn't."

A New Year

"I remember being at Marcia's when Jim called me." I sighed, relieved to have survived the crisis.

"We didn't know what was going to happen." Joel patted Bill's shoulder. "I'm sure glad you made it!"

"Me too! You know, you used to be a head-banger, listening to head-banger music when you were a teen. Now I'm a head-banger too." Bill's humor broke the gloom.

"You're really doing well, Dad."

"Thank you. I praise God that He spared me. We read a passage at Bible study the other night. Do you have a Bible?"

Joel took one from the shelf and handed it to his dad.

Bill flipped through the pages. "Here it is. 2 Corinthians 4:8-10." He read slowly but expressively. "Yes. I was cast down, thrown onto the street, but not destroyed. I almost died but didn't."

Remembering that the Old Testament people built altars in remembrance of significant events, I felt that we needed to somehow seal this date as a blessed date and not a cursed one. "I think we should pray and thank the Lord that Bill is still with us,"

We bowed our heads thanking God for what He had done and asking for guidance in the days ahead.

※

While showering, I thought about the recently completed road work near our house. This project of extending a major highway reminded me of our lives.

University Avenue near our house had already been widened a few years earlier. Now, creeping along behind huge dirt-moving trucks, we saw mountains growing on both sides of the road. One day, the recently improved University Avenue was barricaded to prevent passage. Cars were detoured up, over, and around the imported hills. Before long, the street itself was filled

Bump on the Road

up with dirt as high as the new hills on either side. I didn't understand why they buried this good thoroughfare.

Eventually, it all made sense. Two multiple lane roads evolved overhead. Then dirt was removed from University Avenue, making it useable again. Limited access ramps were constructed on the hill over which we had detoured for a while.

As the perfectly useable road was blocked temporarily by a dirt barrier, Bill's life was put out of commission for a while. He didn't die in the accident, which indicated that God spared him for a reason. Though undergoing reconstruction, God still had a plan for Bill and for us as a couple. What seems senseless to us is an ingredient in the overall plan that only God knows. God didn't cause Bill's accident, but He could redeem it. We were being redirected from where we thought we were going. Because we believed God has a good purpose ultimately, we could trust Him to rebuild our lives correctly.

My hair was full of shampoo when Bill knocked on the door. "It's leaking downstairs. There's soap right below the shower."

"I'm not done! Can't I finish up?" I pleaded.

"Okay, but make it quick."

God, I don't think I can take any more problems! If only Bill could fix things like he used to.

As I dried myself, I heard Bill and Mom talking outside the bathroom. "Look here, Bill. It's this bottle of soap in the closet!" said Mom. "There's a hole in it from a nail and it's leaking all over the place. It must be dripping through here."

"Yeah, that makes sense," said Bill. "This is above where we saw it coming through the ceiling."

By the time I emerged from the bathroom, they had cleaned up the mess and had pounded in the nail. Knowing the truth brought freedom. So often I worry about nothing. This time what seemed complicated had a simple solution.

Till Death

WHILE BILL engrossed himself in computer Free Cell, I sat in bed trying to read before going to sleep.

I felt as though I were a cloth doll with my hair in a child's fist, bouncing along wherever the child went. It was as though I were being dragged from one problem or responsibility to another without rest in between. *Lord, I don't know how much more I can handle. Don't let me fall apart.*

Melancholia began to penetrate as I thought about how I would miss Jody when she moved out.

Lord, You know what is good for me. For us. Thank You that Your plans are good.

At the sound of the back door opening, I donned my robe and went downstairs to see the couple after their movie date.

"How're you doing, Mom?"

I put on a smile. "I'm okay but tired I guess."

Ben cleared his throat and they looked at each other. I wondered what was up.

"We've been wondering if we should wait a little while to get married," she said.

"Why's that?" Maybe she had decided to finish school first. That would keep her here longer.

"We wondered if we should wait until Dad gets a little better." She looked at Ben. "We're concerned about you and don't want to leave you on your own too soon."

Bump on the Road

Would it get any easier to let her go? I could never forgive myself for getting in the way of Jody's life. I took a deep breath.

"That's ... wonderful of you. To be concerned about me." I grabbed Jody with one arm and wrapped the other around Ben's waist and buried my head in the middle of our huddle. Then I let go and stepped back. "The Lord will take care of me. Don't wait on my account."

"Are you sure? We prayed about it and agreed that we're willing to wait." She smoothed my bathrobe collar as she talked.

I nodded. "Grandma's still here. And Peter. I won't be alone. But it means a lot that you would be willing to wait because of me." I needed to keep trusting God with *all* my needs.

April 19 Journal:

God, our completeness is in You for You are our strength in weakness. Thank You that Your plan is greater than ours for Your thoughts are higher than ours and Your ways are greater. You knew about this bump in life's road, this "mistake" even before Bill's conception. This becomes part of who we are. You did not randomly choose to revoke the call on Bill's life. It seems that there will be adjustments to what he planned. I have no idea what's ahead for us, but You know. I have to believe that something better, more effective, more productive in Your kingdom is coming of this.

My husband was determined to drive again. He practiced moving cars in and out of the garage and parking in front of our house. He implored frequently at Courage for another driving test.

After reviewing Bill's neuropsychological exam results, the doctor agreed to let Bill repeat the prescreening. This evaluation showed improvement. They agreed to let Bill take a behind-the-wheel assessment on May 2.

Bill left for Courage full of hope that day but was Mr. Puddleglum when he returned.

Lord, please help Bill find creative outlets of things he can *do now. Help him be patient and find strength and help in You.*

A week later Bill returned home from Courage Center with a glimmer of hope in his voice. "I talked with the man who gave me the driving test. I asked if I could take driving lessons and he said it's a possibility in a couple of months if I continue to get better."

"That's nice." I hoped my husband didn't detect the concern in my voice. I had already explored this option. It wasn't cheap and what if he couldn't drive after investing the money?

Bill's speech therapist recommended Courage Center's Community Reintegration Program (CRP). She said it meets three days a week, six hours each day under the direction of the neuropsychologist. During group sessions, clients work on strategies to compensate for losses, redeveloping social and work skills, and more. I thought it sounded like a good step beyond the adult day program. Bill wondered why it was necessary. He still didn't seem to grasp why he couldn't jump back into life as before.

The last day of May, we revisited another piece of Bill's recovery. North Memorial rehab hosted an alumni tea. We talked with several therapists and our favorite rehab doctor. I was delighted to introduce the real Bill to them—the jovial, friendly, talkative Bill with a twinkle in his eye. They commented on how well he was doing.

Bill agreed to participate in CRP at Courage Center though he seemed perplexed. It was something new. Another adjustment. I attended with Bill his first time, June 5. The day was broken up into several segments which included "Communication and Memory" in a group setting, "Executive Thinking Skills" (higher level thinking and problem solving), and individual time with clients to maintain their planner books. The doctor brought in a life-sized brain model to define and describe the different areas of the brain and what happens during a brain injury.

Bump on the Road

Thanks to Occupational Therapy at Courage Center, Bill expanded his computer usage beyond games. Now he practiced typing and used his new Bible software to read the Bible. I was relieved, especially since we had replaced the old laptop and its outdated operating system.

Another challenge to his previous expertise was the new riding lawn mower. Jody showed her dad how to use it and we turned him loose. Not only did the grass get cut but he also practiced driving. Even so, Mom and I would look at our property and moan over all that needed to be done.

Bit by bit, life settled into a rhythm.

Being without the independence of hopping into his car frustrated Bill. Mom and I either talked him out of it or laid aside our plans. Sometimes it meant a meal in a restaurant or shopping. Other times it was to attend a meeting or conference. Usually I enjoyed the outings but wondered when I would get caught up with to-do's.

Sunday, June 8, six of us stuffed ourselves into my Honda and headed to St. Cloud. A pastor friend had asked Bill to speak at his small church.

Bill described his accident, interjecting humor, and read scriptures which were meaningful to him. Scanning the room, he said, "God has laid hold of me and He isn't finished with me yet. The plan may be different now but I'm leaning on God's grace to accept whatever comes and trust Him."

Many in the congregation were friends. Having prayed for Bill, they commented on his progress.

සො

On a mid-June Saturday, Mom, Bill and I headed out to celebrate a fiftieth anniversary and a wedding. These two events, in

Till Death

opposite directions from our house, would take all day. Burdened by my own challenges to marital bliss, I went begrudgingly.

At event #1, the husband choked up as he thanked his wife for enduring his alcoholism during the first twenty years of their marriage. Sheer commitment had kept them together. I remembered how this troubled marriage was restored through counseling with Bill and Dad Barr at Okontoe years ago. Now, at the fifty-year mark, they renewed their vows and presented new rings to each other. If this woman could persevere, so could I.

From the southernmost suburb of the metro, we drove back through the city and continued a half hour north to Big Lake for our nephew's wedding. The ceremony was tender and sweet. Sitting in the candlelit sanctuary, I remembered my idealism as a twenty-one year old bride thirty-two years earlier.

After celebrating both ends of marriage, I returned home with renewed hope.

Where would I have been if I hadn't married Bill? Knowing how I was, I probably would have chosen a risk-free but dull existence. In spite of our uncertain future, I was grateful for thirty good years together.

Nonetheless, irritations remained. My role as Bill's spouse had abruptly changed. We were no longer equally yoked in life's tasks. Now he was a young teen in an adult body. Self-awareness–understanding of self in relationship with others–was almost nonexistent. He still viewed himself as the middle-aged, educated, intelligent, capable adult to whom others turned for advice and counsel. Now he bristled when I resisted his ideas and didn't trust his judgment. I resorted to devising ways to direct him into what was appropriate. Wanting to avoid arguments or bigger problems, I manipulated and controlled situations.

He couldn't understand why he wasn't allowed to drive a car. "After all, I've had lots of experience driving. I learned to drive in India when I was fourteen years old and have driven ever since." Now my world-traveling spouse couldn't go anywhere alone. These struggles strained our relationship.

I alternated between self-pity and compassion. A severe blow had been dealt to a sharp mind.

We were on different paths, Bill on one through the jumble of injured mind, impaired perceptions, and disabled hearing. Untruths seemed so real and buffeted him mercilessly.

God, You are the God of the impossible. You created his brain originally. Yours is the power to recreate. Your plans for us are for good, not for evil, plans for a hope and a future. You redeem the bad to bring glory to Your name. I lean on You for help.

Two weeks remained before Ben and Jody's nuptials. Would we get everything done?

୨୦

The morning of July 8, 2000 felt like a sauna when Jody loaded her wedding gown into her little red car. "Sure hope it's not too bad out there. I'd feel horrible if someone had heat stroke on my wedding day."

"That storm yesterday knocked out the power but not the heat. At least it's not raining today. I don't know what's worse."

"Me either. Well I need to get going so Julie has time to do my hair. Hope I have everything. Bye Mom."

"Bye. Love yah. Just think, you'll be Mrs. Selin in a few hours." I returned inside, wondering what needed to be done first.

Bill and Josh put on their tuxes and headed out. Before getting to the driveway, they returned.

"These pants are defective. No belt loops so I can't wear a belt to keep 'em up!" Bill gripped the waist of his tux pants. "I'm not wearing them!" He stomped upstairs.

Josh shrugged his shoulders. "Yeah, they fell down."

"Let's try those suspenders that you got for your fiftieth birthday," I said.

Bill moaned. "Those *red* ones?"

"The jacket will cover them up, Dad," said Josh.

I found the suspenders in Bill's drawer and he succumbed to my clipping them to the wasteband. That accomplished, they left again.

Bill still hadn't prepared his wedding message, saying that he would do it on the 45 minute ride to Selins'. Why couldn't he have sat down and done it weeks ago when Pastor Gordy had asked him to?

Jody had been my companion ever since she was a little girl. As I got ready, I remembered her preschool days when she accompanied me to my friends' homes. She would sit quietly by my feet doing puzzles. I loved having her go with Bill and me to India. While Bill flowed with the Indian culture, Jody shared my loneliness in strange places.

She had walked the rugged path of the past year and a half with me. What would I do without her? Thankfully, Mom was still around. So was Peter, our nephew and Joy, our niece, was moving into Jody's old room in the fall. Somehow, by God's grace, life goes on and so would I.

I didn't want to fall apart. Jody deserved a supportive, strong mom.

Armed with umbrellas and hats, Mom and I sat in the kitchen as Angie finished fixing up her tuxedoed ring bearer and his two little sisters. The AC wasn't working in their van so we rolled down the windows, hoping not to blow our coiffed hair.

We arrived as the wedding party posed for pictures in the shade. Jody was gorgeous. A friend had fastened her long hair into a multitude of curls on the top of her head. I wanted to hold my daughter and not let go. But it was too hot.

Bump on the Road

After the photographer finished taking family shots, I went inside where people scrambled at a snail's pace to decorate and set up. I felt awful putting our family and friends through this misery–as if I could do anything about the oppressive heat.

"Oh good. You're here, Cheryl. Where are all the plates, cups and stuff?" Bridget was in charge, but no one had told her where the stuff was.

I couldn't remember but headed downstairs. We had sent everything to Selins' by car loads in stages. After searching to no avail, I panicked. Ben's sister offered to find Marilee.

Soon Marilee followed her daughter inside. "They're upstairs in my bedroom," she said.

Oh. Now I remembered letting that information in one ear and out the other.

Partially unraveled internally, I took Joel's arm as he ushered me to my seat. It felt good to sit.

Pastor Gordy began the ceremony, then gave the mic to Bill. He read scripture and talked about family. I worried about our guests in the heat. Bill's face became as red as the suspenders under his tux jacket. Did he notice the heat as he rambled?

Finally, he pronounced Ben and Jody husband and wife. People gathered about. "It was such a beautiful wedding" from one and "Bill did so well" from another. I broke down and cried in the arms of a friend.

"Cheryl, I'm sorry to bother you." Bill's sister appeared at my elbow. "We can't find the punch stuff." I followed her inside, wracking my brain to remember where it was. By the time I got inside, someone had found it.

Mom persuaded Bill to remove his tux jacket and join her in a shady spot on the porch.

In spite of the chaos, the meal was lovely. A breeze brought relief. Chefs from an Indian restaurant grilled *tandoori* chicken and *naan* (flatbread) on location. This along with salads and wedding cake rewarded our guests' appetites.

After wrestling Joel out of the driver's seat, the just marrieds drove off to begin a new chapter.

Lord, thank You for giving Jody to us for a time. She's not ours to hang onto. She's Your daughter. Thank You for giving her a good spouse and a wonderful extended family.

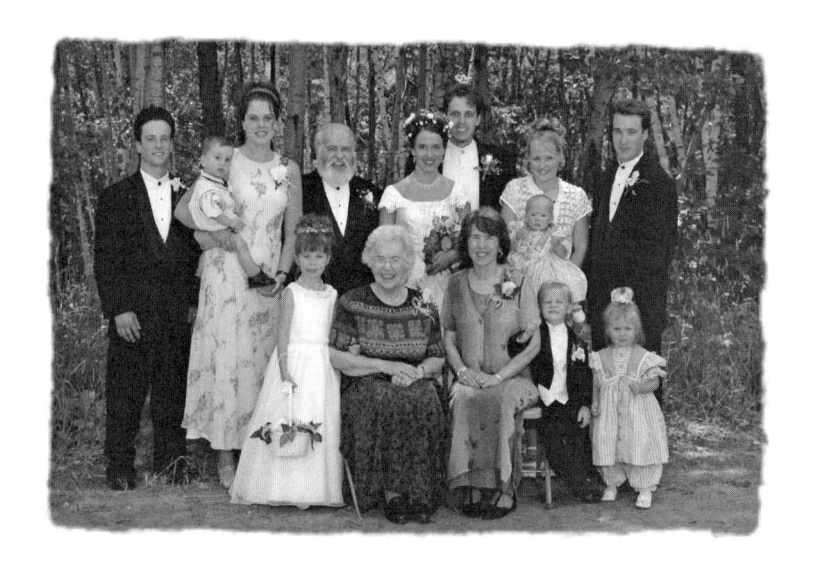

Behind the Wheel

THE NEWLYWEDS settled into their apartment in nearby Anoka. Adjusting to marriage and added household responsibilities challenged Jody as a student. However, she managed to keep her part-time nursing home job, complete her studies, and graduate with her RN degree–pregnant. Once in a while, we talked on the phone and occasionally got together, but it was different. I missed her.

Life settled into a new routine. Three days a week, Bill attended CRP at Courage Center. He seemed to enjoy it and was proud of his accomplishments. His social abilities, including group conversations, improved. He relearned how to use a day planner.

On non-therapy days, I taxied Bill to and from Courage Center for CRP and swimming. One day I talked with Bill's social worker, while Bill looked for the driving assessor. "Bill really wants to drive again," I said.

She nodded understandingly. "It's highly unlikely. I'll talk with him and help him understand."

I was relieved that another with more clout could address this.

Then Bill appeared, smiling broadly. "The instructor thinks I've improved enough that I can take driving lessons, starting in September."

Oh.

Concerned about the cost, I called Courage's driving office. What if we spent all that money on lessons but Bill still couldn't drive? The instructor eased my concerns by saying that he wouldn't be charged beyond the initial exam fee if it appeared that Bill wasn't a candidate for driving.

In September, the man reevaluated Bill's driving and surprised me with his recommendation for lessons. "I believe Bill can master driving again."

We went ahead with lessons.

After the initial sessions, the teacher recommended me to ride along so I could see how Bill did. I sat in the back seat as we looped around the area near Courage. As Bill parked in the underground garage at Courage afterwards, the instructor turned and looked at me. "How did our pal do?"

"He did well," I replied.

"I think Bill will be a safe driver." He patted Bill's shoulder. "Won't ya, Buddy?"

Bill nodded and smiled.

"I'll write a letter to the state indicating that Bill has improved, and to request the reinstatement of his license. I'll recommend that Bill drive with a family member or friend for about six weeks. You'll need to set up an appointment with Bill's neurologist because it's ultimately up to him. If Bill causes an accident, the doc would be in deep trouble."

Turning to Bill, he continued. "Once the state says it's okay, start practicing on familiar roads close to home. I want someone with you at the beginning, too. Okay? When you're more comfortable with things, venture out further." He glanced back at me. "And drive where your wife lets you go."

"Thanks so much for taking the time to work with Bill," I said.

"It's been my pleasure. I tell you what. It's a joy to work with someone with such a great attitude. So many can't drive anymore but they get nasty about it."

Turning to Bill he said, "Before ya' know it, you'll be tooling all over town again." He shook hands with Bill and we climbed out of the car.

Bump on the Road

"Praise God!" Bill's smile was the largest I had seen in a long time.

We met with Bill's neurologist and, a few days before Christmas, a letter came that reinstated Bill's license.

Mid-January, Bill was allowed to venture out on his own within five miles of home, during non-rush hour times, and not on freeways. As he became re-accustomed, he could eventually drive anywhere.

This step toward independence was harder for me than launching our driving teens. His first chance at freeway driving was a Sunday afternoon. I white-knuckled when he cautiously merged onto the interstate. Others whizzed by and glared at us. I worried about being rear-ended. Then I remembered that I needed to trust the Lord. I had asked God to direct through the driving instructor at Courage, hadn't I?

By March, Bill was allowed to drive anywhere, providing that he stayed off the freeways in heavy traffic times. He finished CRP in November but continued going to an optional follow-up group on Thursday afternoons. As part of a vocational rehab program, he volunteered in the CRP office.

Bill improved in solving problems, helping out around the house, sensing the needs of others, tracking conversations, and functioning independently. He even mastered phoning in his prescriptions, using phone key pad and obeying prompts.

Since Bill could now drive independently, my schedule decongested significantly. His geographic awareness gradually returned.

April 14, 2001 Email update:

> Two years ago this Easter, Bill was slipping further and further into a not-so-hopeful medical prognosis. One doctor had told us that, at best, Bill could regain 80% of his former functioning. If we hadn't hoped in the resurrecting, creative power of Christ, we would have crashed

in deep despair. Now we rejoice over continued progress. I believe that we are seeing at least 90% recovery. Bill is beginning to pick up where he left off.

When he learned that Bill was driving again, our Indian restaurant owner friend asked to meet with Bill. My husband returned home that day with a list and enthusiasm to get started. The restaurant needed curtains so I got involved, too. Bill and I picked out the fabric. By driving to three locations in the metro, Bill bought enough matching fabric for the project. I sewed the drapes. Bill bought the rods and hung them.

Our friend asked Bill to make archways like he had done before his accident. Bill rummaged through his materials and found the pieces from the other project to use as patterns. It was a good brain exercise to retrace his creative steps from before. Bill completed the projects, with some help from others. It was more difficult than before, but I was proud of how my husband stuck with it, determined to press through and fulfill his commitments.

Last Sunday night, Bill and I shared at a healing service in a nearby church. That was an awesome experience. Again, we saw how much we have been carried by the prayers and friendship of people all over. A teary-eyed woman came to us after the service and said that she had been a seminary student while Bill was at Bethesda. A pastor friend had told her about Bill and asked her to go there to pray for Bill.

The next day, our pastor friend forwarded an email from her:

> How could this be the same man who never spoke a word to me and could only meet my gaze with a blank, empty, lifeless stare? ... I carried these lifeless eyes in my heart for two years ... burdened over and over again to lift Bill up in prayer. I tried to imagine what his voice

might sound like ... what his handshake would feel like ... what his smile might look like ... and wondered at the beautiful soul that was locked up behind the dark curtain that met me each time I would visit. I questioned how God could possibly rescue this soul so tightly locked up inside the prison of his own injury. As I continue to pray for Bill and his family, I will no longer be seeing the lifeless eyes from the past, but instead I will see the sparkling, vibrant eyes of my brother in Christ.

***

A vocational counselor guided Bill in completing job application forms. By June, he was hired at the airport to assist elderly and handicapped people get to and from their flights. After several delays in getting started, the job settled into a three day per week routine. Bill commuted in heavy traffic at least an hour each way.

Besides working at the airport, Bill picked up miscellaneous projects for Indian friends.

Wanting to explore the possibilities of getting into hospital chaplaincy, Bill met Bethesda's chaplain. He couldn't give Bill a job but encouraged him to volunteer at Bethesda. Upon this recommendation, Bill attended three training sessions.

Because of Bill's increasing commitments, Courage Center released him from his volunteer duties there. Yet, I still worried. On top of full days away from home, Bill worked into the night on restaurant projects. He went from too much down time to not enough. He fought sleepiness with several cups of caffeinated drinks a day.

August 23, 2001 email update:

The neurologist, Bethesda chaplain, and public health nurse have all told us recently that Bill has recovered remarkably, considering how he was during those early months after injury. We covet your prayers for God to bring him into where He intends ministry-wise for Bill's remaining years. The sense of a call to the people of India remains strong within him. How is that to be walked out now? We hang onto the promise that God has a plan for good, not for evil, for a future and a hope.

September 17, Bill underwent a second neuropsychological evaluation at Courage Center. Dr. Norm reported "improving abilities in overall intelligence, auditory memory and attention to the mid-average range or above. Mr. Barr has had more significant improvement in executive skills and visual memory ... truly significant improvement in his ability to do various day to day tasks. Mr. Barr's one remaining area of deficit appears to be in speed of processing, where scores remain in the borderline range .... It is often this area that is hardest to change ... I have had few opportunities to report on such consistent and significant improvement in my experience working with many clients. It is my pleasure to report that this kind, gentle and humorous man appears ready to function at a considerably higher level than was the case at initial assessment seventeen months ago."

The doctor said that Bill would do better in structured situations than in open-ended impromptu settings. I had already noticed this difference between my husband pre-accident and now. He also attributed Bill's success to the CRP program. Though I agreed, I was certain that the multitude of prayers worldwide redirected the path of Bill's outcome.

಄

Chander called me at work September 25, 2001. "Cheryl, Bill had a seizure."

"What?" I didn't believe it.

"He had a seizure when he was at the new restaurant. Pal Cheema called me because he didn't know how to reach you."

Bump on the Road

I called the restaurant. Bill's sister, Mary, was there with Bill so Pal put her on the phone.

"We had just eaten lunch and Bill wanted to take me up onto the roof to show me the project he was supposed to work on," said Mary. "As he was going into the kitchen, he fell on the floor and started shaking and drooling."

"Oh no!" He had a grand mal. "What did you do?"

"We called an ambulance. They're here now, wondering if they should take him to North Memorial Hospital."

"Yeah, he should probably go there. It's close and they should still have his records."

"I'll find out how to get there and drive the car over. Can you meet us at the hospital?"

"Yes, I'll leave right away." I hung up the phone, feeling as though I had been punched in the gut.

On the thirty minute drive to North Memorial, several thoughts cycled through my mind. Why didn't Bill stop pushing himself before it came to this? I'm sure glad it didn't happen while he was driving or on the roof! What's this going to do to the progress he's made?

I didn't know what to expect upon arrival at North Memorial's emergency room.

Bill was fully conscious though sleepy when I entered his curtained cubicle. They had administered medications and run tests. A nurse said that seizures are common for people with traumatic brain injury and can be brought on by fatigue. For this reason, most TBI survivors are kept on anti-seizure medications indefinitely.

Released from the hospital, Bill went home with a prescription for Dilantin and instructions to see his neurologist right away. Gone were Bill's driving privileges. Again. Unless the physician had another solution. Mary drove the Olds home and Bill rode with me.

Behind the Wheel

A week later, we saw the neurologist. Though understanding and sympathetic, the doctor couldn't allow Bill to drive. The state restricts driving for six months following a seizure episode. Occasionally it could be repealed but he doubted that we had grounds for that. He told Bill to stay on Dilantin.

Riding the bus to work would have taken two hours each way so Bill let go of his airport job. He also put most of the projects for Indian friends on hold.

Dilantin dulled Bill and made him sleepy. At first I was glad that Bill was catching up on rest. However, I felt that he was regressing. I asked the neurologist about newer medications that didn't have these adverse affects. He warned that they were expensive but we felt it was worth the cost. Quickly Bill regained the ground he had lost.

Since Bill was determined to paint the restaurant ceiling, I agreed to help it happen. We went at 9:30 p.m. To avoid disturbing customers. The cook gave us some food before they cleaned up. We ate and then got busy. Before sunrise we finished, returned home, and went to bed.

Pastor Gordy asked Bill to do projects at church. While I worked in my office, Bill sheet-rocked and painted a small room. Indian families, who lived nearby, hired Bill for tasks in their homes. Mom and I helped him get to and from.

Somehow we managed those six months of no driving. An appointment with Bill's neurologist in the spring confirmed that Bill was okay to drive again as long as he remained seizure-free. By this time, we had decided he needed a different vehicle than the big brown Olds. Joel located a bare bones panel mini-van for $400. It was ugly but much better for hauling tools and supplies.

Return

THROUGHOUT HIS RECOVERY, Bill's thoughts returned to India. Whenever he brought it up, I groaned inwardly. Bill wasn't aware of the differences between his former self and the one now altered by the accident. His counselor at Courage Center had said that his self-awareness was incomplete, impairing him from seeing what was missing. She said that this was common among brain injury survivors because memory was sketchy. Bill was certain he could travel to India independently as before the accident. I knew otherwise. How could I be honest without devastating him?

I believed that, in the right timing and situation, Bill would go. Marcia, my friend in Holland, had shared a dream of Bill going back but not alone. In her dream, he was being carried by others and would go in a different capacity than before. I wondered who could escort him.

In the fall of 2002, Pastor Gordy's Indian pastor friend, Paul, visited our church. He was spending a few months in the States and invited Bill and me to return to India with him to teach at his Bible school. Since Pastor Gordy knew Paul and had been to his ministry base, he felt that this would be a good test run.

We accepted Paul's invitation and booked tickets for a month in India.

Return

October 17, 2002 newsletter excerpt by Bill

> As the Lord has been healing me, I have had a desire to return to India again to visit our friends and minister there. Recently we have been invited there. For this invitation we are grateful and are now making arrangements. We are planning to go for a month, leaving November 5 and coming home December 4. Cheryl and I are traveling together and look forward to our trip. Cheryl wants to go with me to visit the hospital and the doctors from whom I received surgery and medical care for three weeks. We praise God for my healing and restoration and want to share that with them and our other friends.

We flew into action, preparing to meet Paul in Atlanta to travel with him to his city. I emailed Brother Kaushal and other friends to arrange two weeks in North India after two weeks in the southernmost tip at Paul's ministry base.

I prepared several Bible studies to present while Bill poured over notes from previous teachings, listening to tapes and preparing.

Jody took us to the airport during the first November snow fall. "I wish I could go with you guys," she said. One year old, Audrianna, snuggled closer to her Mama.

"Me too," I said.

A lot had changed in four years. Jody had graduated, become a nurse, and was now expecting child number two. I wondered if and when we would return to India together.

We hugged goodbye and flew into a rainy Atlanta, met Paul and chased him the rest of the way to India. Repeatedly I asked him to slow down and wait for Bill. We landed in Paris and boarded another plane to Mumbai, India. We arrived there at midnight and slept in chairs until time to fly to Kerala before sunup.

Approaching our destination, we traversed between two layers of clouds, with the rising sun casting a salmon colored glow on the cumulus puffs. The scene awed me as much as a world-famous site. Unlike rock formations and mountains, this view was momentary and seen by a few within a window of time. God's boundless beauty is infinite. He paints the big picture of which this was a tiny part.

The first evening at Paul's, I sat on the balcony in front of our upstairs room. The view before me was breathtaking. I watched the clouds get darker as they crept over mountains, rice fields, rubber tree plantations, a river, and a church steeple in the distance. On the immediate grounds below were a large variety of trees bearing coconuts, mangos, bananas and more.

The next day we started teaching. An hour before class, I struggled to put on a sari. I went downstairs to ask Mercy, Paul's wife, if it looked right. She and her helper stifled giggles.

"Let Pria help you," said Mercy.

Pria, the helper, unwound the five yards drooping around my body as I pivoted in the middle of the kitchen floor. I was grateful for the long slip and the blouse which served as anchors for the sari. Mercy handed me a bunch of safety pins. "Hold these."

When Mercy and Pria finished, I was securely wrapped, pinned in a few places, and ready to greet my students.

The next day I tried again. Though better, my wrapping needed adjustment. Pria explained the process as she draped me. The third day, I passed the test. Mercy and Pria nodded and smiled. "You're looking good!"

The fourth day, something went wrong. Class was about to start, but my clothing didn't cooperate. I dashed downstairs to find Pria or Mercy. The place was stone quiet and no one was around. I returned upstairs and started over. *God help me!*

Somehow I put myself together and taught the class without losing my attire.

During the three hour church service Sunday morning, I sat in the back row next to Mercy. Bill sat on the men's side at the front with Joy Paul. The only fan was in the front. I felt like I was going to melt.

Mercy went to the front to speak. Though the female students wore head coverings the whole time, I noticed Mercy let hers slip to her shoulders. If she could go without, so could I. Wrong. She returned to her seat, looked at me and whispered. "You need to cover your head."

Miserably hot, I slipped out to get a fan I had seen in the house. Back in the church, I found an outlet a few feet away and plugged in the fan. One of the young men turned it off and said it was too much draft. Oh.

When church was over, I eagerly retreated to our air-conditioned room.

A few days into our time there, Paul's family started sniffling. "It's the change in weather," Paul said.

Really? I hadn't noticed.

Bill and I each taught a 45-minute session per day. Bill's topic was "Ministering in the Holy Spirit," based on notes he had pulled from his archives. I taught Bible studies on random topics. Some students knew English but others didn't. Interpreters translated for both of us. Bill's typical response to my "How did it go today?" was "Good."

After the hectic days of getting ready for the trip, I relished the slower pace and enjoyed meals with Paul's family. No two meals were alike. Mercy asked me to teach her how to make pizza and cake. We shopped and found most of the ingredients. However, pizza isn't the same without Italian spices and mozzarella cheese.

Bump on the Road

At the end of two weeks in Kerala, we flew north. Brother Kaushal met us at the Delhi airport and took us to their home. "Brother Bill, you are doing well. God is good."

Sona smiled and hugged us. "Praise the Lord. Thank You Jesus."

The next morning, we rode a train to another city for a week with Scott and Anita, our friends who had assisted me on Valentine's Day in 1999.

Though we enjoyed visiting them and other mutual friends, it was not like before. I talked more than Bill did. Scott was busy with his work so we hung out mainly with Anita and their daughters. Scott helped us book train tickets back to Delhi and reserved a room in a downtown hotel for our first night in Delhi. Then we returned to Brother Kaushal's center for a few more days where Bill taught a few sessions at the Bible school.

Bill wanted to see where he had hit the ground so Brother Kaushal took us to the place. For being such a life changing spot, it looked very ordinary. Bill pumped Brother Kaushal for details. We parked and the two men walked down the street. During a lull in traffic, Brother Kaushal walked out to the middle of the road and pointed down. I stood by the car and shot pictures. I wondered what passers by thought of the American taking pictures of the road.

Brother Kaushal's daughter, Vinita, was home from Australia briefly. Aware of our eagerness to visit the hospital, she drove us there. When we pulled up to the front, something didn't look right. We parked, anyway, and walked to the entry that had become so familiar four years before. I talked to a man inside who told us that the hospital had moved and where. Vinita recognized the area and found it quickly.

I was bummed that Bill couldn't see the actual site but hoped that the same staff was there. Especially the doctors.

I greeted the receptionist inside. "This is my husband, Bill Barr. He was in Orthonova January 1999 after being in an accident. I wanted to show him the hospital and see the doctors he had if they're still here. "Is Dr. Sing here?"

"No. He's in a different city."

"Dr. Natan, the neurosurgeon?"

"He finished for the day and went home a little while ago."

This wasn't turning out how I had hoped. I tried again though unsure of the third doctor's name. "Is Dr. Bose here?"

"Yes, come."

She rose and led us past a lobby full of people to a room in the corner. A doctor entered shortly. He looked familiar but I wasn't sure if he was the one I knew.

"Do you remember us? This is my husband who was here for head injury from an accident almost four years ago."

The doctor nodded and shook both of our hands. "Sit here, please."

"We are visiting and I wanted to show my husband Bill the hospital that took care of him. I wanted you to see how he is doing."

The doctor began asking Bill questions about his health. Then he took Bill's blood pressure. I began to wonder if the doctor misunderstood why we were there.

"I just wanted you to see how he's doing since he was still in a coma when we left. I wanted everyone here to meet the real Bill."

The doctor continued asking medical questions. "I want to test his oxygen level." He put a tester with a red light on Bill's finger. "I think you should be tested for sleep apnea. How long will you be here?"

"We are leaving tomorrow to go home," Bill said.

"You should ask for a sleep apnea test." After some exhortations to get more exercise and watch his diet, the doctor stood and shook our hands. "Thank you for coming."

Bump on the Road

As I walked past the front desk to head out, a young man apprehended us. "You didn't pay."

Without argument, I returned and paid the equivalent of $8.50 US. Evidently, they didn't understand our intentions to simply visit.

The next day we flew home, weary but grateful for a good trip. I relaxed, knowing we had negotiated India in our changed form. Even so, our future remained a mystery. Had we accomplished anything significant on this trip?

Subsequently, Brother Kaushal wrote, "Every time I pass by the route, I thank God for the miracle in Bill's life. It is simply the expression of our Father's heart in Heaven that Bill today is glorifying Him every day."

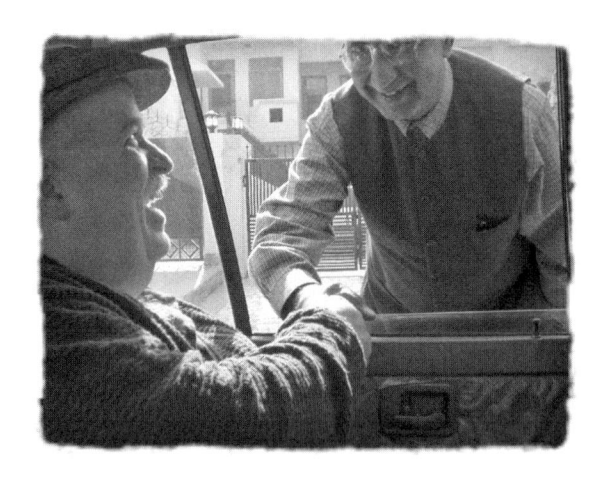

All I Need

ON A CHILLY, fall day in northern Minnesota, family and friends gathered at Okontoe for another wedding. This time it was Mark and Nancy's daughter, Chrissy. Stopping along the way to Okontoe, I had bought a card.

We stayed in a cabin at the south end of camp, a ten-minute walk from the wedding site. At 12:30, a half hour before the wedding, I thought I had plenty of time. Since the reception would be held near our cabin, I decided to leave the gift at the reception site. Bill had left earlier to set up the video camera.

I dragged my suitcase out from under the bunk bed and changed into my wedding clothes–denim skirt and a sweater with a necklace to dress it up a bit. Then I put on my new jacket. It would be perfect for this day of questionable weather.

Grabbing the gift, camera, umbrella, and purse, I crossed the yard set up with picnic tables for the reception and went into the dining hall. *Hmmm, I wonder where I can put this gift so that they don't miss it. Oh, here's a spot by the guestbook...maybe. Wait a minute! They won't know who it's from! I forgot the card. Rats!* My load was starting to feel heavy but I dashed over to where the car was parked several yards away.

I dug past the umbrella, gift bag, and camera on my arm to unzip my purse to grab the car key. Time was ticking quickly. Upon opening the glove compartment, my heart sank. No card. *What on earth did I do with it? I'm getting spacey and I don't like it!*

Bump on the Road

I couldn't remember doing anything other than securing it in a safe place during our trip. Back in the cabin, I rummaged through stuff. I got hot so I shed the jacket. *Lord, where is it?* Not really expecting an answer, I suddenly remembered. Sure enough, the small bag was sitting safely on the top bunk out of reach of small grandchildren.

I sat down on the bed and dashed off a wedding blessing, returned the card to its envelope, and headed back toward the dining hall. *Nuts! Now I forgot the camera!* Back to the cabin again. Then back in the dining hall, I deliberated over where to put the gift, finally placing it on a shelf safe from small hands but still visible. Hopefully.

Now it was almost 1:00 p.m.. If I didn't hurry, I would miss the processional.

Then I realized that I left my jacket at the cabin. *Too bad. I'm not going back now.* I felt my earlobes. I'd forgotten my earrings, too. *Oh well.*

As I approached the wedding site, Chrissy and Pete were hiding behind a tree–that is, from the perspective of most of the guests. I waved and smiled as I walked past them. At least, I didn't miss their entrance!

Skipping the usher protocol, I hastened toward one of the front rows. Bill stood there with a large umbrella over his head and the video camera mounted on its tripod. He was ready for action, looking quite dapper in his wool hat. I scooted behind him and took a seat next to Josh and Angie on a hay bale.

Leaning toward Angie, I whispered. "Have you ever had one of those dreams when you can't find something, you're running late, and you wake up before you get there?"

"All the time," Angie replied.

"I feel like I had one of those dreams except it was real. At least I got here!" *What's my problem? I just had myself to get ready. No kids.*

All I Need

About 250 of us sat on bales of hay facing the wedding "altar" with a glimpse of Arrow Lake behind through the trees. Surrounding us were golds and bronzes against a backdrop of evergreens. Chrissy's desire for fall colors was fulfilled.

I looked at Mom's back as she sat with Nancy in the front row. Seven years after Bill's accident, Mom was now 84 years old. Within a short time, she had grown frail. Earlier in the year, she had fallen and fractured her hip. *Age comes whether we like it or not.*

Sweetness and tenderness flowed between Chrissy and Pete.

Taking Chrissy's sister by the elbow, Pastor Don said, "Annie, please help me with an illustration for a minute. Now lean against me and I will lean against you." Back to back, they leaned against each other. "Chrissy and Pete, you're to lean on each other but not just on each other. If one of you backs off, look what happens." He stepped away. As Annie began to tip, he broke her fall and both chuckled. "Now remember to lean on each other but also on the Lord! He will not let you fall."

"You are to care for each other. Pete, God has entrusted you with this woman to care for and nurture her."

Bill and I used to help each other but what about now? I had become the pillar supporting both of us, but now I felt like I was crumbling.

I can't fall apart. Who would take care of us if I can't?

Could Bill manage if something happened to me? What if he had a stroke or got worse again? *God, I am weak. I need Your help. You are my heavenly husband!*

After I prayed, I felt years of self-effort, holding life together, striving to be appropriate, and perfectionism wash off in waves. *I'm God's child, beloved and cared for by Him. That's all I need. I have fretted about doing everything right my whole life! Instead, God wants me to trust Him as I wanted our children to trust me when they were young.*

Bump on the Road

Fellow wedding guests had also endured recent fiery tests. One woman had come without her Alzheimer's-afflicted husband. Another's daughter had incurred brain injury. *Yes, life isn't perfect. No matter how sincere the marriage commitment, we are human and things happen outside our control. We need the Lord. He is faithful to fill in the gaps. He will take care of us, no matter what. I need to lay down my strivings over finances, time management and relationships.*

It was a new day.

The ceremony finished. Standing and brushing hay from my skirt, I realized that I am simply one of my Father's beloved daughters. Why *wouldn't* the God who created this beauty around us look after me, His child?

I will always have all I need because I'll always have Him.

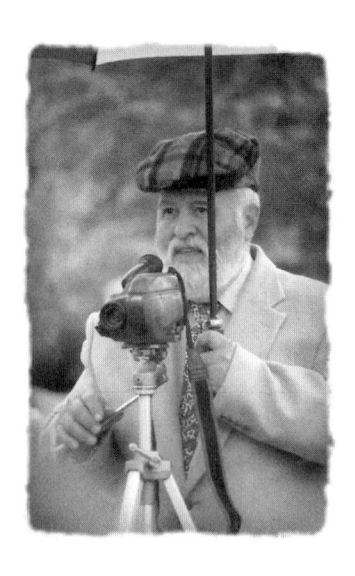

Last But Not Final Chapter

THE PACE OF OUR STORY has slowed to a new routine as we grow in our love and understanding of each other's needs. I'm thankful to have my loving husband back. On Valentine's Day, Bill emerged from his basement office with a typed letter in hand:

I LOVE YOU, VALENTINE CHERYL, MY MATE!!!
February 14, 2004

Dearest Cheryl,

Today as I have been spending time at home to plan this letter, I have been pondering and studying the Bible and what it says in 1 Cor. 13 about love. I have read it in five different versions and they all affirm the facts I know and feel about our love.

In our life together I have known and experienced and still do see and receive love these ways with and from you. Thank you so much for continuing to love all of our family. I rejoice in you and with you as love flows through and to all of our family.

You have had to bear all things, believe all things, hope all things, and endure all things related to my two encounters with death from my head-banger in India and my heart surgery last summer. [Bill had quintuple bypass surgery in June of 2003 and was released to go home three days later. I was astounded by his quick release from the hospital.] Your love shows through each aspect of standing with me and persevering with me through these to healing and renewed life and ministry.

You are so special and I praise God for you and your ongoing love in my life and our family. I pray that His love will break in and upon you each day as you walk with Him and minister. I LOVE YOU AND APPRECIATE YOU MY DEAREST WIFIE!!!!

I am and always will be your ever-loving hubby, Bill

☙

January 14, 2005 Journal:

It was frigid the other night when Bill and I went to Culvers. We had a corner booth and hardly anyone else was there. We talked about various concerns, taking turns initiating prayer about them like former days. The next day, two of our big concerns resolved. We joined forces against our challenges.

A couple of days later, I read Luke 18 where the verse about Jesus and the children arrested my attention. Could my "reality thinking" prevent Bill (and us) from fulfilling God's plan? Maintaining my guardian caregiver role, I repeatedly remind him of "reality," especially in financial matters. Wanting to be a responsible and good "steward" of our resources, I come against his faith on certain things. With childlike faith, he has believed for the impossible. Anxiety and fear have not been an issue for him.

Lord, You know I want to be responsible. But unbelief is sin. So is anxiety. Help me discern the difference. Please forgive me, Lord, for being like the unbelieving ten spies who only saw the giants in Canaan. Instead You desire the faith of Caleb and Joshua, ready to go in and possess the Promised Land. My Promised Land includes complete restoration for Bill, healing from stress of my recent years, fulfillment of

God's plan for our lives, and ALL that we need for current medical and living expenses.

Anxiety, and unbelief have been uprooted in Bill's life. Instead, he has the simple faith of a child. This pleases God far more than striving to be responsible and realistic.

Help me submit my concerns to him in a loving, respectful, wifely sort of way. I need to allow him to come to You as a child but relate to him myself as an adult. He is Your child, not mine.

The phone pulled me from my thoughts. Jody's three-year-old Kaylee wanted to talk to Nana. What an apt reminder to keep my heart soft and trusting like a child's.

ಬಿ

February 13, 2005 Journal:

Lately I've asked Bill for his opinion more frequently. I realized that this is probably the Holy Spirit prompting us to "submit to one another." It is creating more unity between us. We had become isolated and independent from one another through the TBI (traumatic brain injury).

Anticipating Valentine's Day, I realize Bill has been more romantic lately than I've been. He brings me tea in the mornings, bought me expensive heart earrings, brought red roses to work for our anniversary, bought a desk chair for writing, and gave up his office downstairs so I could have art space. Ashamedly I have been remiss in returning romance to him. Forgive me, Lord, and help me. I need to voluntarily serve him rather than having a "serve yourself you lazy bum" attitude when he wants me to get stuff for him. God continues the restoration process with fine-tuning and tweaking, especially in my attitudes.

ಬಿ

Bump on the Road

August 27, 2007 letter from Bill on our anniversary:

> Isaiah 40:27-31 (Assurance of the Lord's help and strength in our life and "work or ministry")
>
> Bill and Cheryl Barr CELEBRATING 39 Awesome Years together as a family and ministry team!
>
> In this 39th year we expect the Lord to do awesome things in and through us in His plans for our destiny. We have talked about some of the things on our hearts for this season of our lives. (mission work; writing; painting; finding His plans for whatever He has in His heart for us to do and be!)
>
> We are aging and getting tired often, yet He reminds us in His Word: those who wait for the Lord will renew their strength; they will mount up with wings like eagles, they will run and not be weary. (Isaiah 40:31) Let us proceed into this new year with His promises!
>
> We are a creative team gifted by the Lord to BE creative. He is the creator of our gifts and abilities and will expand and increase them this year as we wait upon Him! ... We are also the parents of three awesome sons and daughter, and 11 awesome grandchildren. ... God is so good to all of us!
>
> We are pregnant with expectations of awesome things happening this 39th year of our amazing marriage! Some things will take time before they come to "birth."
>
> Prayer: Lord Jesus, we wait upon you as we begin year 39 for You to give us new ways to use Your gifts. Please move by Your Spirit in and through each of us and our families this year to be and do awesome things in Your plans for all of us.
>
> Lots of love, "restored" hubby, Bill

☙

The Last But Not Final Chapter

March 16, 2011 Journal:

I'm seriously considering a different direction for the sage and forest green sweater that I began to knit in 1998. Though it's almost done, I lost zeal when I realized what was involved in making it fit properly. The sleeve would fit a 6'4" man; the torso would fit Jody's nine year old Audrianna. Even if I unraveled it to redo, would I wear it?

In an afternoon, I could use it as fabric to cut out mittens and a hat to sew together on my sewing machine. The more I think about it, the better this sounds. Mittens and a hat would be much more useable. Who knows? There might be enough to make several.

Would this be giving up? I don't think so. Forging ahead stubbornly could be worthless. Change can be a form of acceptance and redemption, converting it to better use. This could be an act of release, letting go for a higher purpose.

Okay, maybe I'm getting too philosophical about this but didn't Jesus use parables to teach lessons?

I see a parallel between this and our lives. The plan Bill launched in 1995 was interrupted four years later. Since then, he's undergone lengthy reconstruction resulting in something different. Is the original plan to be put back together with modifications? Or should the fabric of his life go in an entirely different direction?

ଔ

Following a series of major health issues condensed within a short time, Mom Barr passed away in January 2007. I have been blessed by two wonderful mothers. My mother taught me valuable practical skills during the first 21 years of my life before her death in 1969. Though no one could replace Mother, Bill's mom became *Mom* very naturally. From her example I learned further

Bump on the Road

lessons for being a wife and mother. Both helped me become a woman who loves God.

By this time, nieces and nephews had finished college and gone on. Bill and I became sole inhabitants of our home. It was time and we were ready. Now we're a couple of mid-sixties folks, growing older together.

The pattern of our lives and ministry continues to emerge. When I recently painted a large painting for an Indian restaurant, I tasted how my love for painting could merge with Bill's heart for Indian people. The circle of Indian relationships within our city is still growing larger.

Writing our story has been good for me. It reminds me how far Bill has come from where he could have ended up. In the depth of discouragement during North Memorial Hospital days, I had wondered if death would have been easier. Now I shudder when I realize how close we came to losing him.

Though the accident changed some of Bill's abilities, his personality was protected. I am thankful to have my loving spouse back. It is as though he died and then resurrected. My husband has endured a hardship which would leave many depressed, fearful, angry and bitter. Instead, Bill is cheerful, generous, kind and optimistic.

In subtle ways, Bill continues to improve, despite the counteractive effects of aging. Bill's sister Suzanne commented recently that he seems better each time she talks to him every month or two.

Unlike the first year of his return home, Bill faithfully does his "homework." This includes laundry, washing and putting dishes away, straightening, taking out the trash, and more. There was a time when I wondered if he would remember how to help out. Well, he does and it's wonderful.

The Last But Not Final Chapter

Bill's confidence in God's best for his life has enabled him to embrace the changes. Striving to figure things out has been replaced by simple trust in God.

One Indian friend recently told another that he had been deeply concerned about Bill after his accident but was amazed by how well he has recovered. He also commented that Bill was one of the most honest and kind people he has known.

I'm proud of my husband. When our kids went to Christian school, they received Character Awards at the end of each school year. Thirteen years after his accident, I think Bill should earn Best in Show.

If you're a motorcycle rider and a short, balding man approaches you at a gas station and encourages you to use a helmet, it's probably my husband. Please be patient and understand he's speaking from his own life-threatening and life-changing experience.

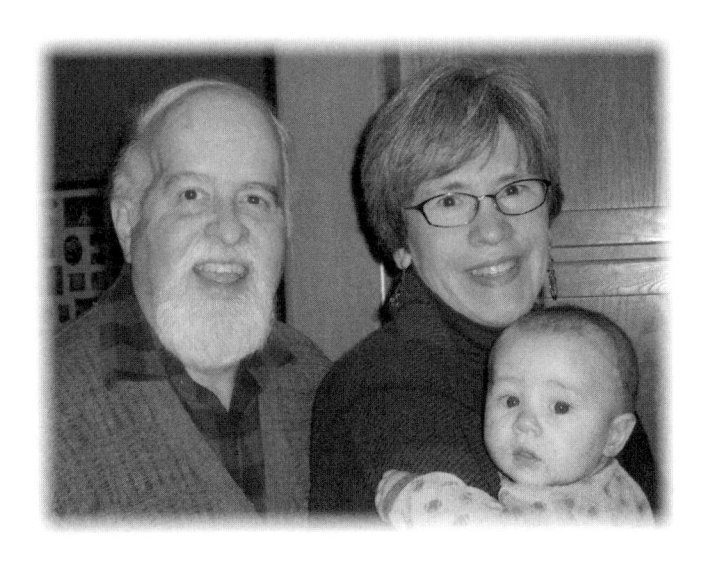

Epilogue

By Headbanger Husband

CHERYL WROTE sharing how God revealed Himself to her and our family through scriptures, answers to her prayers, and the hundreds of prayers of others who received her updates. This is also the first time I read the whole account of my injury and restoration. I learned how severely I was injured and the challenges of finding healing and therapy. In many ways I was distraught about how difficult the process was. My greatest sorrow was for Cheryl and my family and friends as they were so upset with my inability to communicate or do what they or the medical staff wanted and needed me to do. I grieve for her and them for the slow recovery process from brain injury.

What did I feel while my wounded brain slowly began to return to "normal?"

I don't remember anything before Bethesda Hospital. There I was angry when my bathroom was locked. I liked having family and friends visit me. (Now I am very happy to be with my family and friends at home and in their homes, etc.) The programs at Courage Center were rewarding and helpful. Now I like going there for follow-up meetings.

I was happy when Cheryl and I were invited to go to India with Paul to teach, followed by visits in North India. My heart for India and Indian people remains strong.

The Last But Not Final Chapter

Again I continue doing remodeling projects as ordered by my East Indian customers. The process of taking orders and then going and doing the work has helped me heal and learn new skills. The main difference I notice is that it takes me longer to do things. Praise God for His healing!

In 2007 I began working part-time as a custodian and continue this now.

We have led a home group for "empty nesters" for a number of years. We have potluck meals, study the Bible, and pray together. These evenings are wonderful.

We are also a part of a new house-church led by our East Indian friend and his wife. I have helped him do Bible studies and share in the service. I enjoy this group because people from all over the world attend. We sing worship songs in various languages. It is a fascinating global fellowship.

Thank you to all who prayed, loved, cared, and supported us after I severely banged my head. I'm so grateful I'm here and alive!

Bill Barr, October 2012

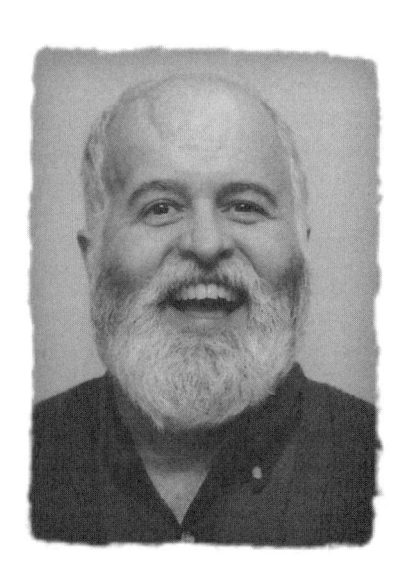